Natural Remedies

Naturopathy Guide To Heal, Protect Yourself From Common Ailments

(Herbal Remedies For Alternative Healing Using Organic Antibiotics)

Jessica Conrad

Published By **Phil Dawson**

Jessica Conrad

Natural Remedies: Naturopathy Guide To Heal, Protect Yourself From Common Ailments (Herbal Remedies For Alternative Healing Using Organic Antibiotics)

ISBN   978-1-77485-871-4

No part of this guidebook shall be reproduced in any form without permission in writing from the publisher except in the case of brief quotations embodied in critical articles or reviews.

Legal & Disclaimer

The information contained in this ebook is not designed to replace or take the place of any form of medicine or professional medical advice. The information in this ebook has been provided for educational & entertainment purposes only.

The information contained in this book has been compiled from sources deemed reliable, and it is accurate to the best of the Author's knowledge; however, the Author cannot guarantee its accuracy and validity and cannot be held liable for any errors or omissions. Changes are periodically made to this book. You must consult your doctor or get professional medical advice before using any of the suggested remedies, techniques, or information in this book.

Table Of Contents

Introduction

In this day and age, many people turn to traditional medicine for their medical needs. Of course, there are often complications associated with these solutions. There are two issues that you need to address. You now have to deal with the first problem.

Over the years, I realized this was a common problem and that many people are seeking holistic solutions to minor issues. This is what motivated me to create this book. I hope you'll find many solutions to everyday issues and live a happier and healthier life.

Chapter 1: The basics of hair loss

Knowing the causes of hair loss is key to finding the best solutions. Hair can be found on nearly all parts of the skin. The exceptions are the palms of our hands and the soles of our feet. The average amount of hairs found on an adult's scalp is approximately 150,000. A typical adult's hair loss per day is about 100. This means you don't need to panic if you notice this much hair on your comb. Because these hairs are so fine, it is impossible to see them with the naked eye.

Each human hair's follicle has a life cycle that includes the three phases anagen (catagen), telogen (telogen) and finalization. As an individual matures, the rate of hair growth slows. Anagen is the stage where hair grows the fastest. This phase can last up to six years. Next is catagen. This transition period lasts two to three weeks. Telogen is also known as the resting time, and it lasts about three months. You'll know when you have a shedding and the new hairs come out. This means that the cycle is back to its original start.

The life cycle for each hair follicle differs from one person to another. It is affected by many factors including climate, age, diseases and many other factors.

Alopecia is scientifically defined as hair loss. The types of hair loss are listed below.

1. Involutional Alopecia. This is a natural process that occurs as we age. Slower hair growth leads to a gradual loss of hair. This is because there are more hair follicles that succumb to the resting period.

2. Alopecia canadensis. This condition can quickly strike children and young adults. The condition can range from a sudden loss of hair, to total baldness or complete baldness. The good news is that approximately 90 percent of those affected experienced normal hair growth within a few years.

3. Alopecia universalis. This is a serious condition characterized by the loss of all hair in the body.

4. Androgenic androgenic alopecia. This is a rare genetic condition that can both affect men and women. This is called male-pattern baldness for men, and female-pattern baldness for women. This happens sooner in men than for women. Many men experience hair loss signs as early as

their 20s. These signs include a receding or completely lost hair at the crown and scalp, as well as a slow-to-slow thinning. Most women notice the obvious signs of hair loss in their 40s, or later. The crown and scalp are the most affected areas.

5. Telogen effluvium. The condition is temporary, and it affects your scalp. This happens when the resting phase occurs and a large number of hair follicles become exhausted. In this case, hair begins to shed.

6. Trichotillomania. This is self-inflicted. This often happens in children. A person suffering from the disorder may pull his/her hair frequently, causing the hair to thin.

Common Causes of Hair Loss

What causes hair thinning? These are some of the most common reasons for hair loss.

1. Genetic composition. This is true for those who are affected by male or female pattern hair loss. This is something you cannot change, but cosmetic surgery can be done if your hair needs to grow back fuller. If you don't want to go under

the knife, prepare yourself to accept that this may happen.

2. Stress. Stress can cause people to lose their sleep, feel irritable, or eat poorly. While these are all signs of hair loss, it is usually temporary or no. While some may believe that hair loss is due to stress, there are very few who actually are. It is part of the stress and torture that they are experiencing.

Emotional stress, such as from heartache or sadness, can lead to physiological stresses. A hormonal imbalance can occur when you seek comfort from food and alcohol after the breakup of your partner. If you're losing your hair more often than usual, it is likely that your physiological changes are to blame and not your partner.

3. Pregnancy and contraceptives. This applies to women that have used contraceptives while they weren't ready to have babies. You'll see a lot of hair fall. You can stop the shedding once you have decided to become pregnant. While pregnant women have thicker hair, it will become thinner and less dense months after childbirth. Hair that has not fallen out during pregnancy may start to shed off. Women who are trying to lose weight

soon after giving birth will notice a greater hair loss. Although contraceptives have a significant effect on many women, it does not always happen to all. Some women may not notice any changes in their hair's growth or hairfall.

4. Hormones. Hair fall is caused by abnormal levels of androgens. These hormones are male hormones which can be produced by both the male and female genders.

5. Fungal infection. Ringworm is the leading cause of hair fall. Ringworm can affect all parts of the body. But, it's more apparent on the scalp. If the condition is severe, patches of hair loss may occur. Tinea capsitis is also known as this condition. This starts as a small pustule that grows in size. It then causes baldness. The temporary baldness occurs because of the fungus entering the hair follicles. Itchy, reddening skin around the hair loss areas is another sign.

6. Drugs and medications. Certain medications can lead to temporary or permanent hair loss. These drugs include birthcontrol pills, medications that control blood pressure, and drugs that are administered during chemotherapy.

7. Too much hair care products and too harsh treatments can cause hair loss. Hair can become brittle if it is allowed to be bleached or treated too often. It can also happen if your hair is not washed enough or you use a blow dryer too often. This can be caused by hot irons, braids, and tight ponytails. Hair fall is caused by scalp damage, but not as severe a as baldness. It is temporary and can easily be reversed by changing hair habits.

8. Diseases. Temporary hair loss could be due to various medical conditions. These conditions include anemia or diabetes.

9. Wrong diet. Temporary hair fall can occur if you don't have enough iron or protein in your system. This can also occur if you have a strict diet.

When is it time for you to alarm? You'll know when your condition is serious and how to treat it.

Chapter 2: How to Stop Sleep-Disrupting Habits

Your current self-help tactics could be making it worse than helping. The long-term effects of using alcohol or sleeping pills to help you fall asleep could make your problem even worse. These activities will disrupt your sleep even more. It will only make it harder for you fall asleep at night when you consume excessive caffeine during the day. Your daily habits could be the key to ending your insomnia. You may find it takes a while for your body adapt to the changes. But once it has, you will feel much more comfortable sleeping.

You can continue recording your insomnia as you did in the beginning. You can also record details from your day and what your sleep routine is. Keep track of how late you go to bed each night and when you wake in the morning. Are you falling asleep where? What have you eaten or drunk during the day? What were your most stressful moments? Jot them down.

Perhaps you've noticed that caffeine intake after a certain time can affect your sleep patterns. You might be amazed at how easy it is for you to fall asleep when switching from evening coffee to herbal tea. It is possible that late-night television viewing may cause insomnia. It is possible to set a time for the TV to go off and instead, read a book. Your sleepless nights could also be made worse by your smart phone, tablet, and laptop. Before you go to bed, turn your device off. These small changes can make all the difference in curing insomnia. You will be able decode the cause of your sleep problems as well as find ways to fix them by keeping a sleeping diary.

Improved sleep can be achieved through the adoption of new habits.

You should ensure that your bedroom is not too noisy, dark, or warm. The outside world, too much light and excessive heat can cause insomnia. An earplug or white noise machine may be useful to help mask outside noises. Darken your room by using shades or drapes. Reduce the temperature of your heater or open your windows a little to prevent your room from getting too hot.

Establish a sleeping schedule and adhere to it. It is important to wake up and go to sleep at the same times every day. This goes for weekends, too. This will help your body to reset.

Avoid taking naps in the middle of the day. Naps make it more difficult to fall asleep at bedtime. Take a 30 minute nap if you are forced to. Avoid napping after 3 p.m.

Avoid doing strenuous or stressful activities before bed. These include strenuous activities, major life-changing talks, arguments and television, computer, or other video games. Instead, read or listen to soothing music. Recharge your batteries and take a deep breath.

Make sure your eReader is not lit up. To make your sleep easier, choose one that needs an additional light source.

The latter half of the day should be avoided. Try to stop drinking coffee and other caffeine-containing beverages if insomnia is a problem. Drinking alcohol in the evening can impact the quality of your sleeping. Nicotine is a stimulant. Avoid smoking before bed.

How to improve your sleep quality by helping your brain regulate itself naturally

Your brain naturally produces melatonin, which is necessary for your body to regulate its sleep-wake cycle. Light exposure is key to melatonin's production. Lack of light exposure throughout the day can make you feel tired. Too much artificial light at nights can reduce the production of melanin, making it harder for you to fall asleep.

To naturally regulate your body and prepare for a peaceful night's sleep, here are some things you can do:

Increase your daytime exposure to sunlight. When you're at work, take a break and walk outside during lunch. Take a walk outside in the sunshine. Let the light in by opening your blinds.

Try to reduce the amount of artificial lights you are exposed to at night. Switch to low-wattage lamps, install room darkening shades in the bedroom, and shut off all electronic devices at least one hour before you go to bed. A sleep mask can be used to create darkness in your bedroom to aid you in falling asleep.

People who work nights and late-night shifts may experience disruptions to their sleeping patterns. If your job requires you be awake at night, you can alter the above sleep habits according to your specific schedule.

Additionally, sunglasses can be used to trick your biological clock and induce sleep. Similar to the above, you can mimic sunlight by sitting in front a bright yellow light source when you wake up in mornings. Keep your commute time to home short as you will be more alert and awake than if it were longer. Even if you are able to adapt to your changing schedule, you should avoid frequent shift changes between day or night shifts to keep some kind of routine. You can also limit the time you spend on your night schedule if it is difficult to adjust to. This will help to prevent mental and physical health problems. Once you are back at home, make sure to close the curtains and turn off all light and sound sources. (If you live in a noisy area, earphones that plug into nothing or even earbuds can be a big help.) To rest peacefully.

Chapter 3: Natural Brews To Treat Coughs And Flus

There are many natural remedies that can help with common cough symptoms. These natural remedies have been shown to work well and can speed up the body's recovery. The best thing? The best part? Many of these ingredients are easily found in every kitchen. Let's get to it!

Thyme - Thyme has been approved by the German government as a treatment for coughs, upper respiratory infections and whooping colds. This is for a very good reason. Do not underestimate these little leaves as they contain countless compounds that are extremely potent in relieving cough. Thyme flavonoids aid in relaxing the ileal, tracheal muscles. This is important when one has a cough. Thyme is also known for helping to reduce inflammation. Mix two teaspoons of Thyme tea leaves with a cup of boiling water. Let it steep for ten mins, then strain the mixture before you drink.

Flax Honey Lemon - OK, it might not look the best but don't let that stop you from using it. Boiling flaxseeds and water in water will make a thick and sticky gel. However, this gel can be very effective for soothing your throat and bronchial tubes. It is possible to make this syrup super-soothing by adding lemon and honey, which act as mild antibiotics. What should you do? You can boil two to three teaspoons of flaxseeds in one cup of water. Let it cook until it thickens. Simply strain it and mix in three tablespoons honey and lemon juice. Use a tablespoonful when you are in need.

Brewed black Pepper - This natural remedy is actually rooted in two very different traditions, New England folkmedicine and Chinese medicine. It's impossible to find anything more interesting than this, right? Black pepper stimulates the mucus circulation and also increases blood flow. Honey can also be added to the mix as it acts as a mild anti-biotic, which can help with cough relief. Make the tea by placing at least one teaspoon freshly ground black pepper in a cup and two tablespoons of honey. Then, boil the water until it reaches a boil. Let it sit for five minutes. Cover the pot with boiling water, and let it stand for 15 minutes. Strain and enjoy the tea whenever you feel like it. This remedy works best with wet, and it is not suitable for dry coughs.

Lemon - Do you want something simple and quick? Although it isn't for everyone, this method is highly effective. Just quarter a freshly squeezed lemon and then sprinkle salty and pepper on the inside. Simple and fast cough relief.

What about the flu, now that we have dealt with the colds? The flu season is real and should be anticipated. What natural remedies do you have to help with this?

Garlic – It is a natural antifungal, antibacterial and immune system booster that can eliminate any disease. You should not cook garlic as it loses its potency. Another option is to make what's known as a garlic shot. Finely mince one or two cloves. Put it in a small shotglass, and you can enjoy it immediately.

Coconut Oil: Most people already know the many wonderful properties of the coconut. Who would of thought that coconut oil could also be used to heal. Because of its high levels of lauric Acid, the oil is very beneficial for boosting immunity and protecting against illness. It can be consumed with food, straight from the jar, or blended into hot tea. Choose your preference.

Fermented Cod Liver Oil- High levels of Omega- 3 make it an ideal remedy for reducing inflammation and improving our immune health. It also contains vitamin A and Vitamin D that can be used in cases of sickness.

Liquid Chrorophyll – Yes, the compound that gives green to leaves. It acts as an alkanizer, making it harder for viruses to survive. Due to its high nutrient level, it can help purify blood. Take about one teaspoon and add it to your water. Then, drink it throughout the week.

Chapter 4: Organic Superfoods - Healthy Food Choices For A Younger You

People who lived in ancient times are known to live longer lives than people today. They can actually live for up to 100 years while still being physically fit and beautiful. Wondering why? The secret is simple, but still very true today: They only eat organic super foods.

What organic superfoods are available to help you have a beautiful, healthy look and feel great? Here are some examples:

Salmon

Salmon is a favorite food among dieters. This superfood can help you have healthy hair, skin, nails, and skin. Salmon is not only delicious, but it's also a great meal that keeps you full for hours. Salmon can be eaten in 2-3 servings per day to meet your essential fatty acid needs.

Acai Berries and Pomegranates

These red-colored fruits contain anti-oxidant properties that can help protect your skin from all kinds of diseases. You can make your skin look more youthful by fighting off the free radicals that can cause premature and rapid aging. They can also increase blood flow to the skin, which speeds up skin regeneration.

Mangoes, Oranges and Kiwis

The common factor in all citrus fruits is their high Vitamin C level. These citrus fruits have a great taste and can help you keep your gums and teeth healthy. A sweet, tangy flavour can also help satisfy your sweet tooth. This means you don't need to crave sugary or unhealthy snacks.

Vitamin C can also stimulate the production of collagen which is known to improve skin texture, elasticity, and texture.

Flaxseeds

These little seeds will help your skin become smoother and more acne-free. Acne breakouts can be often caused by hormonal imbalance, which is due to insufficient nutrient supply. Flaxseeds provide high levels Omega fatty oils that balance estrogen levels. This helps prevent hormonal imbalances which can lead to mood swings, abnormal weight gain, and acne breakouts.

Berries

Feeling puffy and bloated? Berries are the best way to flush out excess fluid from your body. Berries are high in Vitamin C, Vitamin C, Potassium, antioxidants, and minerals. They can help balance hormones and excess fluid. This super food will help you fight the signs of ageing, thanks to its high antioxidant level!

Berries are a wonderful superfood and can easily be included in any meal. It can be eaten either as a dessert. Or you can make it into a smoothie. Consuming berries can help you to feel fuller for longer periods of time and curb your sweet tooth.

Who said that staying young and healthy was hard? Enjoy these super foods and relax!

Chapter 5: Types Of Herbal Medicine Preparation

Many herbal preparations can be used to extract the maximum benefit from herbs. Traditional herbal preparation meant making tea out of fresh or dried herbs. There are now many methods for making herbal medicines.

Herbal Teas

Herbal teas use liquids extracted from herbs to make water. There are many methods to brew herbal coffee. The following are some of the ways you can make your herbal tea.

Infusion. Infusion refers when herbs such as mint and camomile are extracted in hot water by steeping.

Maceration. Maceration is an infusion of plants that has a lot mucilage. After the plants are cut, they are added to water and left to sit for seven hours or longer.

The process of making herbal tea isn't as complicated as you might think. To reap the full benefits of herbal tea, it is essential that you are able to prepare it correctly. Here are the steps required to make tea.

Mix two cups water with one or more tablespoons of dried herb. You can use fresh herbs by using a handful or one-half cup of the herb.

Put the herb in boiling water, and allow it to steep for around 10 to 20 mins.

You can keep the essential oils contained in the tea by using an enamel teapot or other closed container.

Strain the tea and let the herbs settle to one side. This will make the tea easier to drink.

Add fresh or dried herbs to your glass to make it more interesting.

Refrigerate leftovers, as you can reuse the tea leaves later.

Decoction

The process of making decoction is similar in nature to making herbal tea. However, the liquid must be boiled for a long period. This is typically done on plant parts such barks or roots. This preparation is good if you need to use tough plant parts like roots or stems. Here are the methods for making decoctions.

Use a non-reactive, heavy saucepan.

Mix one cup of water, 2 tablespoons of herb mix together.

For 20 minutes, slowly heat the mixture. Let it cool.

Let the mixture sit overnight in the fridge. Strain the liquid before drinking.

Tinctures

Tinctures are alcohol extracts from plants. Infused herbs can be made into spirits like vodka and grappa. The herbs are macerated before being added to the alcohol. They sit there for several hours. Syrup can be described as a type of tincture. It is made by mixing 65 percent sugar with 35 percent water and herbs. It is then boiled, and then macerated for several days to make viscous. Most tinctures are stronger that herbal teas.

It is vital to learn about the most important component in tinctures. The most crucial component of any tincture is its menstruum. It is a solvent that is used for extracting the compounds in herbs. It is used to extract the compounds in herbs. The most commonly used of these three is alcohol, which can be effective at drawing in fats. These are the steps required to prepare herbal oils.

Chop the herbs into small pieces.

Place them in a glass vase and label it with date and herb name.

Make sure to add enough menstruum into the jar so that the herbs are covered.

Cover it with the lid, and keep the jar at room temperatures in a dark place. Mix the concoction at minimum once a day.

You can strain the contents with a cheesecloth after about two to three week.

Allow the mixture overnight to settle.

Place the mixture on a piece if filter paper to clear it.

You should label the tincture, and keep it in cool, dry, dark places.

Topical Solutions

Many people also use essential oils from herbs to their skin. Essential oils are obtained from herbs by distillation. The essential oils can be extracted using different plant parts such as the leaves, stems or roots. It is best to mix essential oil with carrier oil, such as olive or coconut oil, because pure essential oil can cause skin burns. Some examples of topical solutions made with herbal plans are creams. The majority of topical treatments made from herbs are antibacterial and can be used to treat rashes as well as wounds. Here are the steps for making topical remedies using herbs.

Allow fresh or dried herbs to soak for several hours in spring water. Bring it to boiling.

Allow to simmer for about 30 minutes. After that, strain the liquid from the herbs. Let cool the liquid.

Chapter 6: The 40 + Honey Benefits And Uses

Now that we have some knowledge about honey, and the process of making it, we can look at the many wonderful uses and benefits that this golden liquid has.

Honey Benefits and Uses: More than 40

#1 It is good news for your blood. Honey in tepid waters has the incredible effect of increasing the number red blood cells in the body. This can help people suffering from anemia by increasing their blood's oxygen-carrying ability. Honey-based diets can be beneficial for people with reduced oxygen-carrying capabilities. This causes fatigue and breathlessness. It can also help to reduce hypertension which is a serious condition these days.

#2 It works well as a cleanser. The enzymes in raw honey can help keep your pores clear. Honey's antibacterial properties ensure that your skin is free from any breakouts. Add one tablespoon of honey and two tablespoons each of coconut oil to a small bowl. Massage the mixture on your face without putting too much pressure on the eyes. Rinse the face with warm water.

It reduces hangovers. If you feel groggy or have a hangover and wake up feeling groggy, try mixing some honey (around 15ml) and around 80ml of orange juice. You can also add 70 mls of natural yogurt to this mixture and blend it all until you have a very smooth mixture. Consume this mixture and you'll see how fructose (natural sugar in honey) can speed up the liver's alcohol oxidation process, helping you to stay sober longer.

It is rich in essential nutrients. The vast array of nutrients that honey provides is the most obvious reason to include more honey in your diet. Honey provides a wealth of vitamins and minerals, including zinc, riboflavins, copper, magnesium, iron and other nutrients. This makes honey a far better sweetener than sugar, which can only give you empty calories.

#5 It is an excellent energy drink. If you're looking for a quick boost of energy, but not to increase your caloric count, honey is the best choice. You will notice that the fructose in honey quickly enters your bloodstream. This allows you to receive the exact amount you need, while also ensuring you don't consume more that 17 grams of carbs per tablespoon.

#6 Honey is great at treating wounds. Honey is antibacterial as well as antiseptic. It can be very effective when it comes to wound treatment. It is also one of the most well-known wound dressings. Honey can be applied to the area and you'll notice that swelling, inflammation, and even pain will disappear. It's an excellent choice when it comes to treating burns, as it's anti-inflammatory.

#7 This is a good moisturizing mask. To get the moisturizing cream, you don't have to go to the spa. Honey is a good choice to create the same. Because it draws moisture out of the air, honey can keep the skin hydrated for a long time. You can make a natural moisturizer mask by using one teaspoon honey on clean, dry skin. Leave it there for at least 15 minutes. Then wash it off with tepid or warm water.

#8 It can help improve diabetes. Honey is a natural aid in diabetes management. This is because raw honey raises insulin in the body, and reduces hyperglycemia. Just add raw honey into your diet, and watch how it affects your blood sugar.

#9 It fights cold. If you have a cold, honey made from buckwheat is a great way to keep it at bay. The use of a honey syrup like this is proven to be more effective in relieving the symptoms of nighttime colds in children than using the cough syrup sold at your local chemist. In fighting off infection, honey syrup is truly amazing.

#10 It can be helpful to improve your scalp. Seborrheic skin dermatitis causes itching and dandruff on your scalp. Simply mix honey and warm water in a small amount. Apply the solution to your scalp every other days for four weeks. The itching will go away in a few days. If there is hair loss, there will be significant improvement.

#11 You can use honey for your eyes. In treating eye diseases, honey was most effective in the treatment of ancient Egyptians as well as Indians. Honey can be used to treat many eye conditions, including conjunctivitis, redness, itching and itching. It's also known to be an effective way to prevent cataracts. Just mix honey with warm water. After the solution cools down, use it for an eye bath.

#12 It is good for your immune system. Honey's anti-oxidant property makes it a good choice for helping your immune system. Just squeeze half a lime with 1 teaspoon honey and enjoy it. It will improve your immune system tremendously if this is a daily practice.

#13 It can kill resistant bacteria. Sometimes people feel desperate when their antibiotics fail to work. Honey might be the solution they need. When it comes to fighting dangerous pathogens, such as E. Coli or salmonella, medical grade honey can be a real miracle worker. Clinical studies have validated this.

#14 It is good for overall brain function. Honey is rich with antioxidants, which help prevent cell damage and cell loss in the brain. You will have better short term memory if honey is consumed regularly than if you don't. Honey is also known to aid in the absorption of calcium. This is very beneficial for our ability to process information and make decisions. This can be used to help prevent the development of dementia.

#15 It is helpful in digestion. Honey is mildly laxative so it can be great in aiding digestion. You'll find honey is a great way to help things like constipation and gas. Probiotic bacteria found in honey, like lactobacilli and other probiotic bacteria, can also be used to promote digestion. Use honey instead of table sugar to lower the toxic effects that can be caused by fungi.

#16 It reduces scarring. Honey's skin-lightening qualities are known to reduce facial injuries. Its anti-inflammatory as well as antibacterial properties help tissue regeneration and healing. Use a teaspoon of raw honey mixed with one teaspoon of coconut oils to apply the oil in a circular motion on the affected area for approximately one or two seconds. Let it cool down with a warm washcloth. This process should be repeated daily until you get the results you desire.

#17 It improves your sleep quality. Honey is the right remedy for insomnia sufferers. Honey aids in the release of serotonin. This is a neurotransmitter which can improve your mood. Also, the body converts the serotonin into melatonin. Melatonin is an important chemical compound in controlling the quality and length sleep.

#18 It is an excellent treatment for herpes. Honey's high sugar content helps stop the growth microorganisms from your wound. Additionally, honey draws fluids from the wound and releases low levels hydrochloride when it comes into contact. Acyclovir is a commonly prescribed antiviral medicine for Herpes. A study however found that honey was significantly more effective in the treatment of both genital as well as labial herpes.

#19 It can help with weight loss. It can help with weight loss. You just need a honey-based diet to shed those extra pounds. There is an interesting fact: sugar digestion requires a lot more vitamins and minerals than would be helpful in reducing fats. You will see that honey can be used to replace the sugar in your diet. This allows you to retain those essential vitamins and mineral, which are vital for burning fats.

#20 It can be used to remove dandruff. Are you fed up with dandruff and hair loss? Apply honey, 10 percent warmwater to your hair. Rinse after three hours. Its antibacterial as well as antifungal properties will prevent dandruff due to an overgrowth of fungus.

#21 It is a preventative and controlling agent of cancer. What most people are not aware about, is that honey has carcinogenic-preventing and anti-tumor properties, which make it an excellent choice in the treatment and prevention of cancer. It is a smart decision to add more honey to your diet, regardless of whether or not you have been diagnosed with the most deadly disease in the world.

#22 It is a great remedy for ulcers and other gastrointestinal problems. Honey's antibacterial properties make it an excellent choice in treating ulcers and other gastrointestinal diseases. This is due to hydrogen peroxide, which is released from honey. It is interesting that bees actually add an enzyme in honey to release the hydrogen peroxide.

#23 It is a great way to increase athletic performance. We know that honey can be a quick energy boost, but it's also beneficial to athletes. Honey helps muscle recovery after exercise and helps replenish glycogen that has been lost. It is also a good choice if you are an athlete.

#24 Honey may help with seasonal allergies. Although clinical trials have not proved this, honey could help to alleviate seasonal allergies. This is due to its traces of pollen.

#25 It maintains the body's health equilibrium. Raw honey aids in maintaining the body's health balance. They aid in maintaining an alkaline body pH, which is crucial for good health.

#26 It can be used in antibacterial soap. You can prevent many skin problems by using honey instead of regular soap.

#27 This helps to accelerate the growth of healthy tissue. Honey has both vitamin C and amino acids that can help to keep your tissues healthy.

#28 Great for invigorating mornings. You can get a lot of liver glycogen from honey, which is great for giving you an invigorating boost of energy to start your day.

#29 It regulates your body's cholesterol level. You have high levels of bad cholesterol. Increase the intake of honey to reduce cholesterol.

#30 This helps with the treatment of acne. Are you tired of constantly getting acne? Honey can be your answer. You can apply the honey directly to the area. After that, rinse it with warm water.

#31 Honey is a natural remedy for sunburn. Apply honey to sunburns. Your skin will soon heal!

#32 It is helpful in the prevention of aging. Want to look younger? Honey could be what you need to look younger for longer. It contains antioxidants that protect cells from damage by free radicals. This is what causes ageing. You don't need to stress if your diet doesn't include enough fruits and veggies (to get the exact same antioxidants), Just increase your honey intake to get the same results.

#33 It keeps your heart healthy. Your heart's health is something that needs to be taken very seriously, and you can do just that by ensuring that you have a high honey intake that will enable you to keep your heart in good health thanks to the homocysteine-level-reducing properties of honey.

Chapter 7: How to use Herbal Remedies

There are many ways herbal remedies may be used. I've included the basic recipes along with the necessary herbs and the measurements. A chapter will be included in the book that covers common ailments and the herbs that can treat them. This chapter will allow you the opportunity to expand your knowledge on herbal remedies. You can choose your own application form and adapt the recipes with relevant herbs to your treatment.

All remedies can be used fresh or dried, but both work equally well. It is up to the individual to decide which method you prefer. Though I like growing and using fresh herbs, it's not always easy in the British climate so it is beneficial to keep some dried plants around.

Please Note: The term herb can be used to refer to any part of a plant, roots included.

Herbal Tea

Dosages: 1 Adult dose = 8fl.oz. tea. 2 - 4 times daily

You have two options when it comes to making herbal tea.

Herbal Infusion

When you use soft plant ingredients (e.g. leaves, petals and stems), it can be used to make teas.

Herbal Decoction

You can use this to make teas from hardier plants like barks, roots, seeds, stems, and bulbs.

Infusions:

Dried Herbs - 1 - 2 Tbsp per cup water

Fresh Herbs: 2-4 tbsp for every cup of water

Home Made Herbal teabag: 1 cup

Preparation for Infusion

For flavour and fragrance, you can gently crush dried herbs or chop fresh herbs. Boil the water, and let the herbs steep for about 5 minutes. Stir occasionally.

For up to 30 minute, herbs can be steeped.

You can pour tea into cups by using a strainer. Or, you can strain it into a container to let the liquid cool.

To sweeten, add honey or sugar before serving.

Infusion of Herbal Teabags

If you prefer herbal teabags, you can use the same shop bought teabags.

How to Make an Herbal Teabag

For making an herbal teabag, you'll need a square of muslin (or cotton) and fresh or dry herbs.

Place the square of muslin on a smooth surface. Next, place the infusions herbs into the centre.

Take four corners of the Muslin and hold them together. Wrap the herbs within the cloth.

To prevent herbs from fleeing, tie the corners together. Be sure to leave enough cotton for you to safely remove the teabag.

Decoctions:

Dried Herbs - 1 - 2 Tbsp per cup water

Fresh Herbs: 2-4 tbsp for every cup of water

For evaporation, you will need to add 1/4 cup water per cup

Place water in a saucepan.

Reduce heat to a simmer

Stir the water until it is boiling. Add the herbs and stir.

Reduce heat to simmer. Cover saucepan with a lid, and let it sit for between 10-20 minutes.

Strain the tea. Add honey or sugar to taste.

Herbal Ice cubes

Make sure you cool any left-over tea (pre-sweetened). Then, pour it into an ice tray to freeze. These cubes add a refreshing touch to cool drinks, while also providing a therapeutic aid.

Herbal Compress

Making a herbal compress is easy. Simply make the tea, add the herbs and let it steep for a few minutes. After that, soak the cloth in the tea. Wipe the cloth dry.

Although it may seem simple, this is a great way to combine both heat and cold medicinal herbs to treat the problem area.

Hot Compress

Make a warm compress with hot (not boiling) tea. Use it to reduce joint pain, soothe muscle spasms, relax sore muscles as well as tendons and ligaments. Heat opens up blood vessels and increases blood flow. This allows the body and tissues to receive nutrients and oxygen.

Only use for 20 minutes at one time.

If you are suffering from diabetes or poor blood circulation, heat must be avoided.

Do not apply to open wounds.

Do not apply if there is swelling. First, apply a cold compression to reduce swelling. Then apply a warm compress.

Cold Compress

To reduce swelling, bruising, and strains, you can use cold tea as a compress. Cold compresses reduce blood flow to injured areas.

Only use for a maximum time of 20 minutes.

Although it may seem simple, this is an effective way of combining the essential medicinal herbs with heat and cold to treat the area.

Medicinal Creams

Medicinal lotions are a great way to treat cuts and bites as well as skin problems like eczema.

All creams contain a combination of oils, waxes, herbs, and water. Essential oils may also be used to add scent and healing.

Before you start making the cream, make sure you have the oil that has been infused with the herbs. Depending on your method, the process may take anywhere from a few days to several weeks.

Method 1 - Place the herbs you need in a jar. Then, cover it with oil. Keep at least 1"- 2 inches between your liquid and top of the jar. Cover the jar tightly with an airtight cap and keep it in a warm place for 1 to 2 weeks. Strain the herb mixture to get rid of the remaining liquid.

Method 2 - Use a double boiler (or a bowl that is placed on top a saucepan of boiling hot water) to heat the water. Add oil and herbs to the saucepan. Bring water to a boil and then reduce heat to a simmer. Allow to infuse for between 2-12 hours. Strain the oil for any remaining herb residue.

Do not allow the saucepan to boil dry.

Keep stirring the oil/herb mixture.

Do not allow oil to boil. Oil should be kept warm, but not at a low simmer.

All carrier oils can be used to make cream. They all have different therapeutic properties. Almond Oil (Olive Oil), Coconut Oil (Coconut Oil) are the three most used carrier oils.

Olive Oil – Olive oil is a common ingredient in cooking. However, it can also be used to make herbal salves. Olive oil is moisturising with anti-inflammatory and antiaging properties.

Sweet Almond Oil: Packed with vitamins E, B and C, sweet almond oil is a great option for dry skin conditions. It also reduces inflammation and eases muscular pain. This oil is cheap and widely available. However, it should never be used in treating a nut allergy sufferer.

Coconut Oil – Coconut oil acts as a carrier and will nourish the skin. Coconut oil cannot be infused as a liquid. You will need to use method 2.

Beeswax – You can purchase high quality beeswax as sheets, chips (flakes), flakes, or pellets online. Beeswax turns infused oil into an easy-to use cream. Beeswax can also be used as a skin barrier to prevent water from entering the skin and allow the herb oils to penetrate.

Basic Salve Recipe

20g beeswax

250ml herb-infused carrier olive oil

250ml warm (but not hot) water

Directions for the double burner (saucepan & bowl)

Put water in a saucepan. Add the carrier oil to the bowl. Bring water to a boil, and then reduce heat.

Add the beeswax to infused oil. Stir until wax has melted.

Heat off and add essential oils if needed.

Mix well by adding water little by little. The mixture should have a whitish hue and thicken.

Continue stirring vigorously until all the water has been evenly distributed in the oil and wax mixture. After that, transfer to airtight container. Alternately, an electric mixer can be used for blending the water into the wax/oil mix.

This salve will keep for around 6 months when stored at room temperatures.

Herbal Tinctures

Dosages: To be applied under the tongue or diluted with water

1 oz tincture bottle - droppers hold 30 drops = 1/4 tsp

Keep tinctures for children in an empty essential oil container so that only a few drops can be used.

12 yrs. Adult – 1/2 tsp (22.5ml) 2 to 3 times daily

Child between 9 and 12 Years - 1/4 teaspoon daily, 2 to 3 times per day

Child aged 6-9yrs - 24 drops

Children 4-6 years old can have 15 drops

Children 3-4 years old can have 12 drops

Tinctures work in a similar fashion to infused olive oil. But, rather than using oil to extract the healing properties of the plant, alcohol is used. The plant's healing properties, which are absorbed in the alcohol, are destroyed by the use of alcohol.

While vegetable glycerine (or apple cider vinegar) can be used in place of alcohol, these products will not have the same effect as alcohol. I would always recommend using alcohol to prepare tinctures for maximum medicinal effectiveness. Alcohol can be problematic for people with alcohol issues or children.

The neutralization of alcohol

This will allow the alcohol to be neutralized before the tincture is given. To do this, heat the required amount of tincture in hot water. The heat will evaporate the alcohol leaving only the herb. You can either consume it right away or allow it to cool.

Make tinctures with 80% - 100% proof. This is 40 - 50% alcohol. Vodka is the best option as it is close to pure alcohol. Brandy, whisky, and Gin can also be used.

Making a Tincture

Fresh Herbs: 8oz of chopped herbs per 1 pint alcohol

Dried Herbs: 4oz herbs per 1 pint alcohol

Make sure to gently crush/bruise your herbs.

Add the herbs into an airtight container.

Place the herbs in a container and pour the alcohol on top. Be sure to leave at least 1" - 2" between the alcohol & the top of your container.

Close the lid and allow to steep for at most 2 - 3. For best results, shake the herb mixture 1 to 2 times per day.

After steeping, strain the alcohol to extract any herbs. It is best to use cheesecloth, muslin, or a fine sieve. Press the herb residue gently to get rid of all alcohol.

Decant in bottles (preferable with droppers available from pharmacies or online).

Place in cool, dry place.

The shelf life of tinctures depends on how much alcohol is used.

Chapter 8: Your Health

Your entire body needs to be treated as well as your face. There are many things that can cause rough patches in your elbows and knees. Your back can also get acne or dry skin patches. For exfoliation, healing and maintaining healthy skin, scrubs could be beneficial for your whole body.

Take care of your body

For healthy skin, dress appropriately for the season. You can use sun block or sunscreen if the sun is shining on you. Protect your face from the sun by wearing a hat.

Cover any exposed skin in winter to prevent it from becoming frostbitten or windburnt. Both can cause severe skin damage.

You can protect your skin by using a moisturizer on a regular basis. To prevent your skin from drying out, wash it with lukewarm. Your body should be allowed to air dry when possible.

Your hair

It's washed. It's dried. You style it. To make your hair look great, add products to it. This can damage your hair and leave it dry, dull, and split-ends. Hair can become limp from the buildup of products on it.

Try This:

Mix a tablespoonful of conditioner into a cup. Add half a glass of water. Don't stir it. You can just time how long it takes the conditioner dissolve. It takes quite some time, isn't it? You can imagine how much of it stays on your scalp and never ished off.

Here are some ways to get rid of build-up, balance scalp sebum and encourage hair growth.

Consider what residue your hair leaves behind if you use a conditioner. Add gel, mousse or hair spray to make the build-up even worse.

Oily Scalp

2 tbsp Brown Sugar

2 tbsp Lemon Juice

2 Tbsp coconut oil

6 Drops Petitgrain

3 Drops Lavender

2 drops Clarysage

Dry Scalp

2 tbsp Brown Sugar

2 tbsp Lemon Juice

2 Tbsp coconut oil

6 Drops Lavender

3 Drops Ylang Ylang

3 Drops Rose

Normal Scalp

2 tbsp Brown Sugar

2 tbsp Lemon Juice

2 Tbsp coconut oil

6 Drops Petitgrain

Rinsing the Scrub

Now you have the oil in your hair. Now you must break them down before you wash your hair.

2 tbsp Apple Cider Vinegar

2 Cups Filtered Wasser

* Mix together

* Turn your head back

* Slowly pour it out from the front, and let the water flow backwards. This will break down any oils.

* Do not repeat the steps unless absolutely necessary.

* Continue with the rest hair washing steps.

Oily back

1/4 cup Sea Salt

1/4 Cup Brown sugar

3 tbsp of coconut oil

6 drops tea tree oil

3 Drops Peppermint

3 Drops Petitgrain

3 Drops Cedarwood

Dry your back

1/2 Cup Brown sugar

3 tbsp of coconut oil

6 drops of Lavender

3 drops Patchouli

3 Drops Myrrh

3 Drops Geranium

Normal Back

1/2 Cup Brown sugar

3 tbsp Sweet Almond oils

6 Drops Of Ylang Ylang

3 drops of Neroli

3 Drops of Myrrh

Your chest

I'm not referring specifically to the breasts. I am referring to the area below and above the breasts. You can use the scrubs on your breasts. But, you should avoid the area around the nipple. These scrubs can be augmented with a few other items.

Eucalyptus (Eucalyptus globulus)

The essential oil can be used to soothe burns and insect bites.

I Have an Oily Chest

1/2 cup Sea Salt

3 Tbsp Sweet Almond Oil

6 drops of Eucalyptus

3 Drops of Peppermint

Oily Chest II

1/2 cup Sea Salt

3 tbsp Sweet Almond Oil

1 tbsp ground oatmeal

6 Drops of Tea Tree Oil

3 Drops Petitgrain

3 drops of Clary-Sage

Dry Chest I

1/2 cup Brown Sugar

3 tbsp Sweet Almond Oil

1 tbsp Horsetail

3 drops of Eucalyptus

4 drops lavender

4 drops of Geranium

2 drops of peppermint

Dry Chest II

1/2 cup Brown Sugar

3 tablespoons Pure Aloe Juice

6 drops Lavender

6 drops of Chamomile

3 Drops Patchouli

Normal Chest

1/2 cup Brown Sugar

3 Tbsp Sweet Almond Oil

4 Drops of Carrot Seed

4 Drops Petitgrain

4 Drops Ylang Ylang

Regular: Elbows, knees and ankles

1/2 cup Brown Sugar

3 tbsp Sweet Almond Oil

4 Drops Ylang Tlang

4 Drops Lavender

4 Drops Rose

4 Drops Geranium

Elbows, knees and ankles-scaly

All of us have experienced hard, almost callous-like skin at our elbows and knees. The combination of essential oils, herbs, and essential oils can be used to soften and heat the skin.

1/2 Cup Brown Sugar

2 tbsp Pure Aloe Juice

1/2 tbsp. Kelp

4 Drops Lavender

4 drops Chamomile

2 Drops Petitgrain

* Warm to slightly above the body temperature.

* Apply while it's still warm

Knees and elbows-dry

1/2 Cup Brown Sugar

2 tbsp Pure Aloe Juice

1/2 tbsp. Kelp

4 Drops Carrot oil

4 Drops Frankincense

Arms and Legs-Dry

1/2 cup Brown Sugar

3 tbsp coconut oil

4 drops Peppermint

4 Drops Clarysage

4 Drops Rose

Arms and Legs-Rashes

Sometimes you might get rash spots around the bends of your knees or elbows. Here are some suggestions for what to do if you have rash patches around your elbows and knees. This is for regular rashes.

Recipe I

1/2 cup Brown Sugar

3 Tbsp Coconut Oil

4 drops Patchouli

4 Drops Rose

4 Drops Geranium

Recipe II

1/2 cup Brown Sugar

3 tbsp Sweet Almond Oil

1/2 tbsp Tumeric

4 Drops of Carrot Seed

4 drops Frankincense

4 Drops Ylang Ylang

Cellulite Scrubs

Instead of listing essential oils I can add to the list, let me simply say citrus oils like grapefruit, lime, or even lemon. They all help tighten skin by stimulating blood flow and preventing lymph accumulation.

Cellulite is a form of fat that makes your bottom and legs look like cottage cheese. In an effort to make their bodies look thinner, many people spend thousands each year on cellulite removal. Some people exercise their cellulite off at the gym while others have liposuction done to reduce it. Although exercise is a great way to reduce cellulite, these scrubs can make it even more effective.

Recipe I

1/2 cup Brown Sugar

3 tbsp Sweet Almond Oil

1/2 tbsp. Kelp

8 drops Grapefruit

4 Drops of Peppermint

4 Drops Chamomile

Recipe II

1/2 cup Brown Sugar

3 tbsp Sweet Almond Oil

1/2 tbsp. Kelp

8 drops Lime oil

4 Drops Grapefruit

4 Drops of Peppermint

Recipe III

1/2 cup Sea Salt

3 tablespoons coconut oil

4 drops Lemon

4 Drops Grapefruit

4 Drops Lavender

4 Drops Petitgrain

Chapter 9: Mental, & Neurological Remedies

Anxiety

Anxiety is not as easy as feeling anxious and fidgety. High cortisol levels and insomnia can make it worse. The following natural remedies can help with insomnia.

Chamomile tea. Chamomile is mentioned quite often in this book. Take chamomile or decaffeinated tea to ease anxiety and insomnia.

Omega-3 fatty acids. These fatty acid, found in salmon and tuna fish, can help reduce anxiety. You can also purchase oil capsules to get it. It should be taken in no less than 2.5mg daily.

Passionflower. As a natural sedative, it has been used for centuries in different countries as an anxiety remedy. You can relax and get restful sleep by taking a teaspoon of this herb and steeping it in a cup boiling water for approximately 10 minutes. You should drink this 30 minutes before bedtime. Be aware that you should not consume this if youre pregnant.

Lavender. Lavender is a soothing herb for the eyes as well as the mind. Lavender's natural properties help reduce stress and calm nerves. To induce a relaxed state, you can either inhale lavender oil or diffuse diluted lavender oils into your home.

Mild depression

Many people instantly think of medications and doctors when they hear the word depression. If you have the answers you need right now, you don't necessarily have to resort to medical drugs. You can find these natural remedies in the following list. It is important to address depression by increasing serotonin levels. This hormone has been called the "happy hormone".

Pumpkin seed. Pumpkin seeds have three essential substances that reduce depression: fats (the good kind), magnesium and Ltrytophan. They all work together to keep the brain's chemical equilibrium in check and increase the levels of serotonin. Keep depression at bay by eating a large amount of pumpkin seeds daily.

Chamomile is a tea. This book also includes peppermint and ginger. Chamomile is a common choice because of its many health benefits. As in anxiety, chamomile is good for sleeping problems. Enjoy a warm cup of chamomile about half an hour before you go bed to help relax and promote a peaceful night's sleep.

Green tea. Green tea. Green tea is better than chamomile, so have it with breakfast.

Banana. This fruit is a great way to increase serotonin. While bananas are rich in serotonin (which is what they do), it doesn't actually affect the brain. Your brain will make more of its own serotonin because of the high Vitamin B6 content. Eat it once per day, and preferably before your meals. You can also have it with mackerel or spinach in your meals, since they contain high amounts of B Vitamins.

Insomnia

Insomnia can become a problem when it affects the physiological health of a person or when it hampers normal day to day functioning. It isn't a single condition. Insomnia can be associated with or a symptom for other illnesses like anxiety and depression. It is possible to find treatments that can be applied to insomnia using the same remedies for these conditions.

Melatonin. Melatonin regulates your sleep patterns or your 'circadian rhythm. While there are many available melatonin supplement products on the marketplace, there are natural sources that can be derived from plants. These include feverfew or fenugreek seed. You can have feverfew tea (recipe under the Headache section), 30 minutes before you go to bed.

Tart cherries. Tart cherry is another product from plants that can increase brain melatonin. You can take it in juice or as a beverage, around a glass, two times a day. One in the morning, and one 30 minutes before bed.

Valerian. Valerian, especially its roots, has been used for sedation and sleeping aids for a long time. Therefore, it can also be used to treat anxiety. Valerian root can also be taken in capsules, or as a hot tea. Simply let the dried root in a cup of boiling hot water steep for at least 15 minutes. Strain, then let cool down for 30 minutes.

Chapter 10: Herbal Syrup Recipes

If you have ever made cocktails in your life, you will know how to make herbal syrup. The two main ingredients are water and sugar. Both are common items that all people have access to. This chapter contains a variety of herbal syrups that can be made to make you feel better.

Simple Herb Infused Syrup

What's in the deal?

1 C. water

1 C. Sugar

Options:

5 fresh basil sprigs

Four fresh rosemary sprigs

1 handful mint sprigs

6 fresh Thyme sprigs

8 bay leaves

Saucepan

Cheesecloth

Funnel

8-ounce glass jars and bottles with lid

How it is made

Rinse herbs of choice.

Bring water to boiling. Add sugar to the water and whisk until sugar dissolves.

Pour in herbs. Let boil for 1 minute.

Reduce heat, and let herbs steep in water for half an hour.

Take out the herbs and remove them from the syrup with a slotted teaspoon. Allow to cool.

Spread the cooled syrup onto cheesecloth.

Close the jar or bottle with the label. Keep it in the refrigerator

Lavender Syrup

What's the catch?

A few drops purple food coloring

2 tbsp. fresh lavender blossoms

1 1/2 C. sugar

1 1/2 C. Water

How it's made

Mix all the ingredients together in a large saucepan. Heat at low heat. Stir, and let sugar dissolve completely.

Bring to boiling point and let simmer for 5 min.

Turn off the heat and let it cool for half an hours.

Turn heat back on and bring it back to boiling point.

Place cheesecloth in a container or bottle with lid.

Conifer and Wild Berry Tonic Syrup

What's in it?

1/4 C. vodka, brandy or rum

1 C. raw honey

5 C. water

1 tsp. fennel seeds, allspice, cinnamon, or cardamom

Dried orange peel

3/4 C. mixed herb

2 C. mixed hawthorn berries or rosehips

2 1/2 C. mixed needles for conifers

How it's made

Place plant material in a small pot. Add water until the water is absorbed.

Bring to a boil and then simmer. Allow the liquids to simmer for at least 4 hours, or until they are 1/4 of their original volume.

Strain plant matter using cheesecloth.

Add honey to the remaining liquid.

Stir until warm. Let stand for 10 minutes.

Heat should be removed and the mixture allowed to cool down.

Add your alcohol. Stir well to combine.

Fill into a glass. After storing, let cool.

Elderberry Syrup

This homemade syrup will prevent you from getting the flu.

What's the deal?

1 C. raw honey

1/2 tsp. 1/2 teaspoon whole cloves (or clove powder)

1 tsp. 1 tsp.

2 tbsp. fresh or dried ginger root

3 1/2 C. Water

2/3 C. dried elderberries

How it's made

In a large saucepan, combine water and ginger, cinnamon, ginger, or cloves.

Heat to boiling. Then cover and reduce the heat. Keep the liquid in the saucepan for about 45 minutes to an hr, or until it reduces to approximately half of its original volume.

Remove heat and allow it to cool.

Strain the mixture into a bowl with cheesecloth or a strainer. Strain liquid.

Get rid of elderberries.

Add honey to the mixture once it has cooled. Stir to combine.

Once honey has been incorporated, pour the mixture into a container and cover it with a lid.

Keep in the fridge

Mint Syrup

What's the deal?

2 tbsp. Lemon juice

4 C. water

3 C. sugar

2 C. Mint leaves blended with 2 C. Sugar

How it's made

Bring sugar, water and salt to a boil

Mix the chopped mint leaves once they have been boiled.

Cook for 15 Minutes

Stir in lemon juice.

Allow to cool.

After cooling, cover the bowl with cheesecloth. Then strain the mixture.

Finally, add the mixture to containers that you prefer and seal them with a lid.

Miracle Homemade Cough Syrup

What's in it?

1/2 tsp. cayenne pepper

1/2 tsp. 1/2 tsp. cinnamon

2 tbsp. Honey

2 tbsp. apple cider vinegar

4 tbsp. 4 tbsp.

How it's made

Place all components in a mason pot.

Keep lid closed tightly

Mix together.

Consume 3 tablespoons liquid in the beginning, then continue to eat this mixture all day.

Ginger Syrup

What's in the deal?

1/2 - 1 C. sugar/ honey

2 C. water

1 cinnamon stick

1 C. Sliced fresh ginger root

How it's made

Mix together water, honey, cinnamon, and ginger in a saucepan

Bring pan to boiling point.

Reduce heat and simmer the mixture for between 30-45 minutes to reduce liquid by at minimum half.

Take the mixture and strain it using cheesecloth

Let syrup cool. Stir in honey (if used) until combined.

Use lids of your choice to place in container. Keep it in the refrigerator

Rose Syrup

What's in the deal?

200 ml of water

200g goldencaster sugar

Petals in a deep red rose scent

How it's made

Place sugar and water into a saucepan.

Turn heat up to medium-low until sugar dissolves completely.

Add rose petals. Allow to simmer for 30 minutes.

Strain into an airtight container. Allow to cool down before using.

Lemon Verbena Syrup

What's in it?

1-2 C. lemon verbena leaves

2 C. sugar

1 C. water

How it's made

Take stems out of the leaves.

Bring water to boil. Pour in sugar, stirring till dissolved.

Pour over leaves. Let cool.

Strain into a glass or container with lid.

Wild Cherry Bark Syrup

What's in it?

1 tbsp. 1 tbsp.

2 C. organic zahăr

.5 ounces of herbs of choice

Wild cherry bark:.5 ounces

1 C. organic Cherry Juice or Water

How it's made

In a saucepan, boil water and add cherry bark and herbs.

Strain and discard the herbs.

Mix the cherries with sugar and lemon zest in a large saucepan. Let the mixture simmer for about half an hour.

Allow to cool, then fill the bottle with water. Keep it in the fridge for at least 6 months.

Elderberry Syrup

What's in the deal?

1 tbsp. Grated ginger

5 cloves

1 cinnamon stick

1 C. raw honey

2 C. water

1/2 C. dried elderberries

How it is made

Combine water, berries and spices in a large saucepan. Heat to boiling, then reduce heat. Allow liquid to simmer for 20-30 mins until it drops to half the original volume.

Strain through cheesecloth.

Mix in honey.

Let cool. Let cool for about two to three weeks.

Respiratory Syrup

What's in the deal?

1 C. raw honey

1 tsp. 1 teaspoon

2 tsp. dried elecampane root

2 tsp. dried mullein leaf

2 C. water

How it's made

In a small bowl, mix herbs and water.

Heat to boiling, then reduce. Let cool for about 10-20 mins, until liquids are half-boiled.

Strain into bowl.

Let cool.

Mix honey in the sauce once it has cooled.

You can pour syrup into any container you choose.

Take 1/2 teaspoon for each use.

Keep in the refrigerator for at least three months.

Mint Syrup

What's the deal?

1 C. water

1 C. Sugar

1 C. chopped rosemary leaves

How it's made

Bring sugar and water to boil.

Next, add in the mint leaves. Allow to simmer for 15 more minutes.

Remove leaves and strain syrup.

Allow the mixture to cool before pouring into containers with lids or bottles.

Allow to chill for up 2 months

Elecampane Syrup

This syrup aids in the healing of infections by settling the lungs.

What's in it?

Elecampane Tincture - 1 oz

3/4 C. local Honey

2 1/2 C. Water

2- 3-inch cinnamon sticks

1/2 C. dried Elecampane root

How it's made

Take the cinnamon sticks apart.

Heat water, cinnamon sticks and Elecampane roots to boiling point.

Reduce heat until it reaches a simmering point. Reduce heat to a simmer, stirring occasionally, until liquid is half the original volume.

Strain mixture into a cheesecloth.

Allow honey to cool.

Let it cool to room temperatures, and then add Elecampane.

Mix everything together.

Iron Building Syrup

This iron-rich syrup is full of vitamins and minerals. It will make you feel amazing!

What's in the deal?

1/2 C. dried dandelion leaf

1/2 C. dandelion root

1/2 C. burdock roots

1/2 C. yellow port

1/2 C. nettle Leaf

1/2 C. raspberry leaves

12 C. water

2-3 C. raw honey

7 tbsp. Black strap molasses

4 ounces of brandy

How it's made

Bring water, roots, & leaves to boil. Lower heat, then reduce heat and let mixture simmer until half of its original volume.

You can strain the herbs using a cheesecloth.

Refill the pot with any liquid left over. Allow to cool.

When the mixture is cooling, stir honey and molasses together. After the mixture has cooled, mix honey and molasses together. Stir in well to ensure that it is fully incorporated.

Mix in the brandy and stir.

Keep refrigerated. Consume 2-6 tablespoons. daily.

Persistent Cough Syrup

What's the deal?

7 dried coltsfoot berries

3 handfuls licorice root

2 1/4 C. Water

1/2 C. raw honey

Chapter 11: Natural Remedies For Inflammation

It can be a problem for friends and family members who are experiencing pain or inflammation. It can also make work more difficult and leave you unable to focus. People who suffer from chronic pain are more likely than others to develop other psychiatric symptoms including anxiety and depression.

There are both over-the–counter and prescription medicines that can be used to relieve pain and provide temporary relief. But they may not be the best long-term solution and regular use can be dangerous for your body. What can we do? Natural remedies are the best. Many herbs supplements provide similar relief but do not have long-term side effects.

Let's have a closer look.

Capsaicin

This component is derived from hot chili peppers. It does this by reducing the levels of the P substance that is responsible for the pain. Capsaicin can either be taken in pill form or as an addition to your diet. You can add more hot chili peppers into your meals.

Turmeric

Studies have shown that turmeric's antiinflammatory properties are comparable with Motrin and Hydrocortisone. But, it doesn't cause any side effects. Do not use this herb if you are pregnant or have gallstone problems. You should also consult your doctor or herbalist to ensure the proper dosage.

Basil

This aromatic herb, often used as a garnish to salads or pastas, can provide a potent remedy for inflammation. It can prevent the enzyme from causing the problem. This is very similar to Tylenol and Ibuprofen. It is much more pleasant to eat and has very low risk of causing damage to the organs.

Boswellia

This herb is frequently used in Ayurvedic medicine when treating joint pain and relieving inflammation. It works because the herbs contain components that can reduce cytokine which causes chronic inflammation. There is a possibility of skin rash, but it is best to consult your physician before using it.

Cinnamon

It's hard to resist the cinnamon smell and taste. There are many health benefits to cinnamon, which you will surely enjoy by adding it to your coffee or baking any type of pastry. Its ability decrease the body's inflammation is one of its greatest benefits. It can also reduce the associated pain. Take caution, cinnamon can be very spicy.

Guggul

Ayurvedic Medicine uses this herb to detoxify and relieve pain. In a matter of months, Guggul may also be used to treat knee osteoarthritis. One thing to keep in mind when using this botanical is that it can cause blood clots so don't take it with other similar-acting medications.

Chapter 12: Parts Of The Gi Tract

The digestive system includes several organs. They include the mouth (esophagus), stomach (food tube), small and medium intestine, glands liver, gall bladder and pancreas. The glands produce digestive juices that contain enzymes. This chemically breaks down food into smaller molecules. The digestive system is responsible for providing nutrients to the body and also separates from and discards waste products when food is eaten.

In reality, the digestive tract (GI) functions as a long muscular tube and food processor. The GI tract is responsible for the digestion of food. However, it can also contain toxins. Toxins could include, but not be limited to, food pesticides or specific foods (like Gluten) that can trigger a reaction from your GI tract.

Congenital Defects

Sometimes life throws a curve at us and we are given imperfect anatomy. The function of any of our digestive organs may be affected by malformations. Most congenital problems can be fixed by surgery. If there are any defects in the palate or orofacial lip, this should be addressed within the first three month of birth. Infants born with a cleft palate or lip may have difficulty breastfeeding or formula feeding. These special bottles direct the formula's flow to the back and are used for these cases. There are many congenital disorders that could be caused by the birth of a child, some which require immediate surgical treatment.

Digestive Disorders

Our evolutionary history clearly shows us that we were in the past primarily herbivores. Today, we are omnivores. This means we eat both plant and animal food. These are the facts about our past.

*Human saliva is rich in alpha-amylase. This enzyme is designed to help break down complex carbohydrates and create sugar compounds.

*Our teeth were designed to extract vegetable matter from the ground and grind grains.

*The so-called "canine teeth" aren't like the canines of larger carnivores, such as cats, dogs or canines. They look more wedge-like.

*The human digestive tract is complex and slows down food processing to get all the nutrients.

*True carnivores are quick to digest their flesh.

*Carnivores can eliminate high levels of cholesterol by eating a variety of foods.

*Carnivores lack alpha amylase in saliva.

The result of the changes in our diets over the past 100 year has been the following:

Heartburn is a common problem in America.

*30% suffer from dyspepsia.

*5% of the American populace suffers from peptic Ulcer.

Gastrointestinal Symptoms

The GI Tract has five basic symptoms. These symptoms are often associated with dietary difficulties or food allergies. If you have serious GI Tract symptoms, it is crucial that you consult a physician. This will allow you to rule out more serious GI Tract disease. The chosen physician should be experienced in dealing with dietary concerns and food allergies. We will discuss each of these symptoms and offer suggestions for natural remedies.

*Nausea (and Vomiting)

*Bloating

*Constipation

*Diarrhea

*Abdominal pain

These medications are covered by over-the counter drugs that have a multibillion dollar market. Nearly every hour, a commercial airs for an antacid and similar products on television. This book will provide you with some options for pharmaceutical or natural solutions.

Chapter 13: How to Treat a Cold

Last chapter, we discussed arthritis, a very common disease in older people. Here we'll talk about something more common - colds. You can get them from many different viruses or bacteria but they all have the same symptoms: sore throats, running noses, general discomfort and temperature.

Andrographis

It is a useful herb and is found in the Indian subcontinent of America. It is used by Ayrveda. Ayrveda was an Indian system of healthcare that existed around two thousand five hundred years ago. It has antispasmodic as well as antiperistalsis properties.

This herb is well-suited for treating a common cold due to its many unique properties. Its antimicrobial activities have been promising and it is used to treat colds. The herb strengthens the immune and may reduce the need for antibiotics.

The preparation is very simple. First boil one cup water in a saucepan. Once the water has boiled, add it to the cup. Place the dried adrographis in a tea ball, and then pour it back into the cup. After ten to twenty-minutes of steeping, you can easily remove it. The licorice root can be added to the cup to help reduce bitterness. It is a natural sweetener. You should finish the recipe by drinking the cup without any food in your stomach.

Angelica root

This one is closely related with the Dong Quai. It is one the most well-known Chinese tonics for women. Angelica can be used to induce labor, and to expel the baby's placenta. This is why pregnant women should not use this remedy. It can be dangerous.

It also relieves pain and delays menstruation. This recipe is for women, as many of you know. There are many issues that can occur when the menstrual cycle is disrupted due to a cold. This herb helps to ease the process. It also has a number of other benefits, including reducing congestion and easing fever. It can help with colds and coughs by stimulating the lungs.

It is now time to learn how to prepare it. You need to use the whole plant: the roots, the stems and the fruits. The most common part of the medicine is however the resinous roots. You can use the fresh, dried roots as a decoction. They can also be made into oils. This plant is easy and simple to look after. This herb is easy to care for and can be prepared in a variety of ways.

Anise seed

This herb is often used to make cough syrups. Many people know it because of its sweet and licorice flavour. The seeds and the essential oils are the most important parts.

It was used for gas pains and constipation for many years in North America. It can also be used in colic or rheumatism. The alpapinene and creosol, which are modern medical methods to relieve congestion and ease the symptoms of coughing, provide the healing power of this herb. You can use this herb without the need to mix any chemicals with it. This is a big difference. It also kills germs while clearing your lungs from the effects of coughs.

It can be used as a sweetener in teas, cakes and other cooking. The herb can be sprinkled on cookies and cakes to increase your health. It can be found in many Chinese or Japanese recipes as an ingredients, so you have a lot to choose from when it comes this particular remedy.

Astragalus root

The Chinese medicine remedy huangqi uses the name of this root as both a botanical and English name. It is used for fatigue, lackluster appetite, excessive sweating and general conditions.

Another reason is that Astragalus has a very useful effect on strengthening the body against viral infections, especially when it concerns the heart or respiratory tract. It stimulates interferon formation, which is the key reason for the relief. It is a herb that is very good for the hearts and has scientifically been proven to have a positive effect on the general state of the body.

It can be used to make tea, especially when it is in capsules as an extract. It can be ground into a powder that is very sweet and used to flavor foods and shakes. Chinese medicine experts recommend that one should consume nine to fifteeng per day. This is equivalent to three to five tablespoons of the herb. It is best to make a tea by boiling the dried root with water for a few minutes.

Chapter 14: The Proper Treatment of Hair Loss

The health of your hair is determined by what you eat. In addition to having a good hair-care routine, you should also eat healthy.

Here are some foods you can eat to treat hair loss

1. Prunes. Iron deficiency may cause hair loss. Prunes contain high amounts of iron. The iron deficiency causes hair to become fragile and thin. Hair will fall easily after being combed. Some hair might also become discolored. You can eat a handful prunes as a dessert or snack to increase your iron intake.

2. Carrot. Carrot is well-known for its eye health, but the rich source of vitamin A in it is beneficial for the hair and scalp. It strengthens and shines hair by nourishing the scalp. This will result in less hair falling as each hair will have a stronger grip on the scalp.

3. Almond. This is a good source for iron, Vitamin E and other proteins. This is a better alternative to lower cholesterol. Almonds won't cause hair loss, and can even help prevent it.

4. Oats. Oats are rich in magnesium, phosphorous, potassium. Combining these three elements together will make it easier for you to fight hair fall and help your mane grow.

5. Chickpeas. Chickpeas will help you grow your hair easier if you eat chickpeas regularly. Chickpeas can be a good source of vitamin B6 or zinc. This will help to get rid dandruff from your hair, make it healthier, and prevent hair fall.

6. Raisins. Eaten raisins will increase your body's iron levels, which can lead to the production of hemoglobin. The oxygen is carried to the entire body by the latter, which includes the scalp. When this happens, hair grows better and is prevented from falling.

7. Roast beef. This is a good source of vitamin B6, protein, and zinc that can all be beneficial for your hair. It is safe to consume this supplement in moderation daily.

8. Soy beans. These beans are a great source of iron as well vitamin E. They can both promote hair growth and fight hair loss.

9. Fish. This is a great source of vitamins, which are vital for keeping your hair shiny and healthy.

10. Orange. This orange has a high Vitamin C level that aids in the absorption of iron from other foods.

Important Diet Tips

Your body needs the right vitamins and mineral to prevent and treat hair loss. Here is a list to help you plan your daily menu.

1. Protein. Protein makes up more than 90% of your hair. Hair loss could be caused if there is not enough protein. It is important to limit your intake of dietary protein. It can have a different effect on hair and may even cause other health concerns.

2. Vitamin C. Vitamin C. The body needs Vitamin C to improve its health, stamina, and overall well-being. This is necessary for the formation of collagen. It supports each hair follicle as well as the functioning of the scalp's blood vessels. Your body will absorb iron faster and more effectively if you take this vitamin. Iron is needed to prevent and treat hair loss. Vitamin C when taken in combination with vitaminE is more effective in providing healthier skin and scalp.

3. Vitamin B

Complex vitamins such as B vitamins can be found within the same food items or ingredients. Healthy hair requires a good intake of vitamins B3, niacin or pantothenic Acid, B5, or pantothenic acid. B6 or piroxine. B7 or biotin. B9 or folate. B12 and riboflavin are also important.

Vitamins B5-B7 are helpful in slowing the process of hair color loss and hair discoloration. Vitamin B6 helps in the production and maintenance of melanin. It gives color to hair. This helps to absorb zinc into your body and can also be used to treat hair loss. B vitamins help form hemoglobin. The latter is critical in ensuring that oxygen from your lungs is transported to all of your body tissues, including the hair.

4. Silica. This is also known by the name silicon dioxide. It is vital for the growth and maintenance of the skeleton. It must be present in hair to prevent baldness. This mineral can be found among many foods including red and yellow peppers, beans, green peppers as well as strawberries, cucumbers, asparagus, cucumbers, and potatoes. The amounts of silica present in these food items will vary depending on where they were grown. It is highly recommended to

buy organic varieties that have not been processed.

5. Vitamin A and Beta Carotene. Vitamin A aids in hair growth by making your cells and tissues healthier. Insufficient vitamin A can lead hair loss, and even hair thinning. Beta-carotene acts as a precursor to vitamin A. It contains antioxidants and can be used to make the hair healthier. This ingredient is also found in fruits like mangoes, melon, and green vegetables.

6. Copper and zinc. Copper does not require high amounts. However, supplying the body with a low amount of copper can help the body to perform its functions. This can increase hair thickness and volume. Zinc, on other hand, aids in the production cells, including those found in the hair. Both must be taken in equal amounts. Toxic copper intake can cause liver problems, and zinc excess can hinder the body's ability to absorb copper. Sesame seeds provide a good source for both copper and zinc.

7. Iron. This helps to deliver oxygen to your scalp. Hair loss may result from iron deficiency. It is more common in women at the end of their menstrual cycle, who are also more likely to

experience hair loss. You can ensure that your body gets enough iron by eating foods rich in it such as tuna fish, egg yolks oyster, whole grain liver, whole grains, liver, dried fruit, and lean red meat.

Your hair will be healthier if you plan your meals properly and follow a healthy diet. It's important to know what foods to choose and what vitamins and minerals you should be looking for when grocery shopping, or when dining out.

Chapter 15: Hypertension and The Dash Diet

The Dash Diet, also known to be Dietary Approaches that Stop Hypertension is used for controlling and/or lowering high blood pressure. This diet contains foods and ingredients with low sodium content. This diet includes foods that have been shown to lower blood pressure, as well as being high in nutrients (calcium and potassium) DASH Diet has a lot of fruits and vegetables. It also includes nuts, lean proteins, whole grains. poultry, fish, and other healthy foods. It does limit the consumption of sugary drinks, red meats, sweets, and red meats.

DASH Diet Benefits

Following the DASH Diet eating pattern will reduce your sodium intake. By limiting your sodium intake, you can lower your risk of developing high cholesterol. You can lower your blood pressure if you already have high blood sugar. You may even save your own life by following the DASH Diet, since high blood pressure can lead you to serious health problems such as strokes or heart attacks.

Caffeine & Alcohol

Because caffeine's effects on blood pressure are still unclear, the DASH Diet isn't concerned with caffeine. Studies have shown that caffeine does increase blood pressure temporarily. People with high blood pressure should seriously consider reducing their intake of caffeine.

An excessive intake of alcohol can raise your blood pressure. The DASH Diet has a limit on the amount of alcohol you may consume. I can have no more that one drink per day for women and two for men.

Weight Loss

While the DASH Diet can't be used to encourage weight loss, it could be used in your weight management strategy. You might consider reducing the DASH Diet's daily calorie limit from 2,000 to 1,600 per day. You have the option to adjust the DASH Diet to suit your individual needs.

DASH Diet Meal Plan Sample #1

These are just some of the meal plans you might be able to create with the DASH diet.

Breakfast: 1 small whole wheat bagel with 2 tablespoons decaffeinated peanut butter, 1 orange, and 1 cup fat free milk

Lunch: Spinach salad made with 4 cups baby spinach leaves, 1/3 of a sliced pear and 1/3 of slivered almonds. 1/2 cup mandarin Orange, 2 tablespoons reduced-fat wine vinaigrette. Twelve reduced-sodium white crackers with 1 cup fat-free dairy.

Dinner:Two ounces of herb-crusted, baked cod, 1/2 Cup steamed fresh green bean, 1/2 Cup brown rice, and 2 teaspoons trans fat-free margarine.

Snacks: Four vanilla wafers with 1 cup low fat, cholesterol-free yogurt

DASH Diet Meal Plan Sample #2

Breakfast: 1 cup of oatmeal made old-fashioned, with 1 teaspoon cinnamon and 1 slice whole-wheat toast, with 1 teaspoon transfat margarine and 1 liter fat-free milk.

Lunch: Tuna salad made from 2 tablespoons fatfree mayonnaise, 1/2 c unsalted tuna (about 3oz), 15 grapes, 1/4 c diced celery, 2 cups romaine and 2 cups of lettuce. Eight Melba toast crackers with 1 cup fatfree milk.

Dinner: Beef and vegetable kebabs with 3 ounces of lean meat and 1 cup each of cherry tomatoes, peppers and mushrooms. One cup of cooked wild rice, two pineapple rings and 1/2 cup nuts. Cran-raspberry-infused sparkling water mixed with 4 to8 ounces of cranberry juice.

Snacks: One cup light yogurt with one peach

DASH Diet Meal Plan Sample #3

Breakfast: One cup chopped fresh fruits (such as bananas or berries), topped with 1/3 cup low-calorie vanilla yogurt and 1/3 cups walnuts. One muffin made from bran, with 1 teaspoon of trans-free milk. One cup of fat free milk and herbal tea

Lunch:Curried Chicken Wrap made with 1 whole wheat tortilla, 2/3 cup of cooked chicken (about 3.0 ounces), 1/2 c chopped apple, 1/2 teaspoon curry paste, and 2 tablespoons fatfree mayonnaise. Half a cup baby carrots raw and 1 cup fat free milk

Dinner: One cup cooked whole wheat spaghetti with 1 cup of no-added sal marinara sauce. Two cups mixed salad leaves topped off with 1 tablespoon lowfat Caesar dressing. One whole-wheat bun topped off with 1 teaspoon trans-free Margarine. One sparkling water and one peach.

Snack-Trail mix of 1/4 cup raisins, 1 ounce unsalted mini Twist pretzels, 2 tablespoons sunflower seeds and 2 tablespoons chocolate chips.

Chapter 16: Magnotherapy

Magnotherapy, which dates back more than 6,000 years, is considered one of the oldest types of medicine. It is recommended by doctors as well as physiotherapists, chiropractors and veterinarians.

Magnotherapy: Can it Cure Everything?

Magnotherapy may be the best thing from nature, or it could be akin to Voodoo. It all depends on who you ask.

People think only of herbs, plants, food stuffs when talking about "natural remedies". Magnets are very rarely mentioned. They are powerful, effective and far-reaching.

Although this is not intended to be a review of any company, it is meant to help people with problems with their health. Bioflow is the name that stands out in this industry. Ecoflow, a British firm, makes this product. (http://www.bioflow.co.uk). I do not receive any commission and do not work for them.

Although the company itself is not very nice and their customer service is unprofessional, the products and services are exceptional and comparable to anything else. I recommend that you just put up with them and enjoy their bracelet.

Magnotherapy's history

Magnotherapy, formerly known as MFT (Magnetic Field Therapy), dates back more than 6,000years. This makes it one of oldest forms of medicine. NASA discovered it and made it available to astronauts. Since then, the healing properties of Magnotherapy have been more widely known among civilians. (NASA discovered adverse reactions due to the magnetic force leaving the earth, which was when magnotherapy returned to focus.

There are many options for magnetic bracelets that claim to do different things. These can range in price from just a few bucks to over 100 dollars, and as with most products, you get exactly what you pay.

The less expensive magnetic bracelets may be able to do something but they are limited in their capabilities. However, the Bioflow Elite bracelet is capable of doing a lot and can do almost everything. Ecoflow offers a wide range of

Bioflow Bracelets, but the Elite has the magnetic fields that are opposite. The magnetic force is pulled through the vein by this placement.

Customers with high blood pressure medication have purchased this bracelet, and they have stopped needing it (under their doctors instructions). Others who have low blood pressure medication have stopped using it as well.

Simply put, a magnetic bracelet makes your body perform better.

How Magnets Impact Our Body

A magnet is an element strongly connected to electricity.

An atom has a mass (the nuclear nucleus), and one to several orbiting electrons. The nucleus and electrons each have their charges and their magnetic fields. A new magnetic field can be applied to an atom to move the electron's orbit. This will promote greater molecular bonds, i.e. The exchanging and/or using of electrons.

Without electron movement, changes in matter (water and blood as well as fuel) are impossible.

Electric communication is a vital part of the human body. For this reason, electrolytes are required to send data around the body. The pH, or the balance of acids/alkalis, is a key component to life and pain. The ph, which is responsible for haemoglobin oxygen and circulation, is also important. Magnotherapy is a way to help electrolytes get the right information and maintain a balancedPH.

Electromagnetic machines are used by health professionals to treat patients with a pulsed electromagnetic field. These machines can only last a few minutes and are very heavy.

A Bioflow bracelet with a CRP module creates an electromagnetic field that produces a similar effect, but it does not emit any electromagnetic radiation. It can be worn and carried for indefinite periods of time without side effects. Bioflow magnets are considered a "Class1 medical device." This rating refers to any side effects and class1 is considered the lowest. This means that there is no significant negative side effect.

Central Reverse Polarity

Ecoflow plc has patented CRP magnet technology. This creates a distinct magnetic field, which replicates the pulsed magnetic force generated by electromagnetic generators.

Central Reverse Polarity has been designed to move electrons. Any matter that passes through a CRPF field is subject to an additional "kick", three opposed directional forces. The efficiency of molecules that have been exposed to a CRP fields is higher. CRP modules can have a field which is concentrated in one direction but shielded from the rear. This gives a concentrated field.

Bioflow states that products may take upto three months before they start to work. In fact, they offer a 90 Day Money Back Guarantee for customers who do feel no benefit after that time, less a 15% handling charge.

Doctors, physiotherapists. chiropractors. Veterinarians. Sports people.

Notice: Pacemaker users should not use or wear a magnet close to their device as it may damage it. Use a magnet only around the foot or lower leg.

Even though doctors don't agree on this, some experts believe south pole magnets can accelerate growth of cancer cells. Therefore, it might be a good idea to avoid either bi-pole or southpole magnets if you are suffering from this condition.

Magnotherapy helps with health problems

Magnotherapy has been proved to be helpful in some health problems

Aging – Encourages enzymatic activation which may slow down the aging process. Magnotherapy was shown to increase lifespan in animals according to studies.

Alzheimer's Disease

Antimicrobial - Can fight viruses, bacteria and fungi along with a host of other germs

Arthritis. The "Journal of Rheumatology", November 1997. P. 1200. "Magnetic therapy might be the most effective method to alleviate arthritis pain." "Ecoflows' Bioflow CRP was the therapeutic magnetic magnet (in the shape of a bracelet) used in the trial that recorded a "beneficial impact." It was conducted by a team at the Peninsula Medical School.

Asthma

Bronchitis

Cardiovascular/Coronary Heart Disease

Carpal Tunnel Syndrome

Central Nervous System Disorders: Dr. William Philpott believes in magnotherapy, which can reduce hallucinations or delusions, seizures and panic attacks.

Circulatory Problems

Depression

Dermatitis

Diabetes

Enhanced Energy

Epilepsy

Fibromyalgia

Headache

Healing - tissue and bone healing

Increase sports performance - This is a technique that has been used for many years on racehorses. Bruce Davidson sent his horses to Equine Therapy Center Camden, South Carolina to receive magnetic therapy.

Hepatitis

Inflammation

Lou Gehrig's Disease

Joint pain

Kidney problems

Multiple Sclerosis

Muscle Massages

Nerve damage

Neurological Disorders

Osteoporosis

Pain Relief: Studies have shown that this will help reduce or ease pain and discomfort in a variety conditions including arthritis and fibromyalgia.

Parkinson's Disease

Post-Polio Syndrome. Studies in a placebo-controlled, double-blind study revealed a reduction in pain. Results are published in the November 1997 issue of the "Archives of Physical Medicine and Rehabilitation".

Rheumatoid Arthritis

Sleep - hence, the magnetic pillows

Stress Reduction

Surgery – Studies have shown that healing can be speeded by using a magnet one to two weeks before and after an operation.

Tendonitis

Tourette's Sindrome

Ulcers

The following examples include doctor's views and reports. However, it would take too long to include all of this information with every item on the list.

Important to note is that patients sometimes feel their symptoms increasing within the first twenty four to forty eight hours. This is normal since parts of your body that weren't getting enough blood are now working overtime. This can be solved by wearing the magnetic for short periods of time in the beginning. Then, gradually, you can use it full-time.

Another possible side effect is "cold like" symptoms. These symptoms are caused by the toxins in you body. It is important to drink lots of fluids as these toxins can quickly pass out in your urine. Most cases will resolve in a matter hours with a couple of large glasses of water.

Many prominent institutions, such as the British Medical Journal (December 2003), Imperial College London and Yale Universities, have found evidence that sustaining magnotherapy works in many conditions.

Chapter 17: Natural Remedies For Anxiety

There's always something to worry over, such as money, family, or job. Anxiety seems to be a part of most people's daily lives. However, it doesn't have to make you miserable or keep you from living your best life. You can use natural, safe remedies instead of taking medication. While many of these remedies work immediately, others may help reduce anxiety over time. These lifestyle enhancements will help improve your outlook and life quality.

Chamomile

Chamomile tea has a relaxing effect, and it is often recommended to be taken before bed. Compounds found in chamomile can affect the brain receptors in the same way as Valium, an anxiety medication. It is possible to drink chamomile in tea form or as a supplement. According to results from an eight-week University of Pennsylvania Medical Center study, patients with generalized anxious disorder (GAD), had significantly lower anxiety symptoms when taking chamomile supplementation. A recommendation for anxious days is to consume up to three cups of tea each day.

Regular Exercise

Studies show that as little as 21 minutes a day of exercise is enough to improve anxiety symptoms. You'll feel better about your self and your heart rate will go up. This will send endorphins running through your body. Endorphins play a major role in the body's ability to block pain signals and create a feeling of euphoria. Many scientists believe that increasing your body temperature by exercising helps to alter the neural connections that control brain function. In turn, your body responds by increasing your mood, increasing relaxation, and alleviating anxiety.

The Great Outdoors

While it might seem ridiculous to claim that sunbathing helps reduce anxiety, the truth is quite real. In as little as 15 minutes each day, you can increase the amount of Vitamin D and decrease anxiety symptoms. Japan found that people who spent twenty minutes walking in wooded areas were less stressed than those who did the same in urban areas. Walk around your neighborhood or park for a bit. This will help you be healthier and happier.

Diet

Studies have shown anxiety can be caused by alcohol, caffeine, or added sugars. In addition, anxiety symptoms are also linked to low levels of Vitamin B12, Zinc and Magnesium. The bottom line is that your level of anxiety can be directly affected by what you eat. Therefore, it is crucial to pay attention to what you eat at every meal. Studies have shown that anxiety may be linked to digestive problems. It is important to avoid eating processed and fried foods. An anxiety attack can be caused by waiting too long for food to arrive.

The following foods have been proven to reduce anxiety:

Blueberries

Peaches

Whole grains

Avocados

Oranges

Dark leafy vegetables

Dark chocolate

Salmon

Walnuts

Flaxseeds

All of these foods contain nutrients which help regulate hormones, blood sugar and other body processes to reduce or eliminate anxiety symptoms. Vitamin B, C and Omega-3 fatty oils rich foods are essential to decreasing anxiety levels and improving mental health.

Mindfulness

Because it requires patience, the most awareness and the most practice, this may be the most difficult of all natural treatments for anxiety. Mindfulness, a form mindfulness, is a meditation that comes from the Buddhist tradition. It has been shown to reduce anxiety. It is about paying attention to what is actually happening and not worrying about the future. If anxiety is a constant companion, it's easy to lose control of your thoughts and begin worrying about the future. Instead of allowing anxiety to take control, try taking a few deep, cleansing sighs and considering the likelihood that your fears might come true. It is very unlikely that you will experience a catastrophic outcome if your anxiety is under control. You are less likely to experience a devastating outcome than you think. In reality, there are very few events that can change your life.

Chapter 18: Natural Remedies For Gastrointestinal Ailments

Your stomach and intestines are part of your gastrointestinal tract. The upper tract comprises your stomach, duodenum and stomach. The smaller tract contains your large intestines and small intestinale. Your digestive tract releases hormones such gastrin, secretin, ghrelin and secretin that aid in digestion.

Normally, it takes 30 to 40 hours for digested food through your colon or large intestinale. The digestion cycle is complete when the food has passed through. It is essential that you take care of the gastrointestinal system. A poor gastrointestinal health can lead to serious conditions such appendicitis and abdominal tumors. This could mean that you will need to have surgical procedures.

But not all gastrointestinal issues require immediate treatment. There are natural remedies available for problems such as constipation or irritable intestinal syndrome.

Cranberry juice, such as, can be used to treat urinary tract infection and gastric ulcers. Aloe Vera gel can also be consumed if you have an irritable intestinal syndrome (bloating, gas, diarrhea, and/or abdominal discomfort). Different types of tea can be used to treat stomach cramps or indigestion. Green, mint, ginger and fennel can all be used to reduce flatulence and stomach gas.

Chamomile is a natural remedy for many stomach and digestive problems such as constipation and irritable stool syndrome. Chamomile can be consumed as a tea or as an herbal supplement. Other oils that can be helpful include geranium and peppermint.

Peppermint oils are useful for releasing stomach gas and treating stomachaches. They also help with irritable bowel syndrome, bowel spasms or stomach pain. Geranium oil on the other side can help to eliminate intestinal worms. It can also help with stomach ulcers and duodenal problems.

If you have not used barks before now is the best time to start using white oak and slippery maple. White oak bark has natural antibacterial qualities that can be helpful in eliminating parasites, preventing infections, and keeping them out of the gastrointestinal tract. Slippery-elm bark has soothing qualities and is helpful in treating gastritis.

Roots are good for the digestive tract. For instance, Dandelion root can be helpful for digestion and can reduce constipation. Chicory root helps detoxify your body, regulates your metabolism and purifies your blood. It can also help with colitis, gastritis, hemorhoids, and other conditions. It can help prevent and remove intestinal worms.

Your stomach can damage your gastrointestinal cells more easily by stimulating the production of mucosal tissues in your digestive tract. It's also useful in reducing stomach and intestinal inflammations. Ginseng has many uses that are popular in Asian cultures. Ginseng can be used for many purposes, including to improve your immune system, digestion, lower cholesterol levels, prevent cancer and other health benefits.

Additionally, spices can be used to treat various digestive disorders. Garlic can also be used to treat gastric and duodenal ulcers, fungal infection and stomach viruses. It can also help with intestinal parasites. Turmeric or curcumin has anti-inflammatory property, which allows it to reduce damage done to your gastrointestinal tract by polyps.

You can also use cayenne pepper as a preventative for gastric and duodenal ulcers. Apple cider vinegar is also a good option to fight infection, prevent indigestion and treat heartburn. To combat Escherichiacoli and to stabilize your blood sugar, you can also use cinnamon.

Chapter 19: Different Forms Of Taheebo

Taheebo is readily available in many forms. It can be taken internally via tablets, capsules. Liquid extracts, tea powder, and tea, or externally as salve. There are many places you can buy taheebo, such as online sources, health food stores, and drug stores.

Manufacturers have different recommendations on how much taheebo they recommend. The recommended dosage is different for each manufacturer. To release active ingredients, practitioners recommend that the bark is simmered or cooked for approximately eight to ten minute. Others believe that it would work better if the bark is soaked, rather than boiled. The soaking process takes longer than boiling and preserves the natural elements which could otherwise be destroyed by heat. The bark of the tree can be used in either of these ways. Taheebo comes in packets as "loose bark". People buy the bark and make tea with it.

Also, it is wise to be very careful about what brand you buy. Some brands of taheebo are able to deliver noticeable results while others may not. Some brands sell taheebo, but the capsules only contain the Pau d'Arco bark. This is often considered almost useless.

Vibrant Life is a popular Taheebo variety. Because it is extracted differently, it is claimed to be superior than competitors. The bark is then soaked using a mixture glycerin/alcohol, which are good solvents and effective at extracting active ingredients from the bark. The bark residue mass is then strained and left as a liquid, which contains alcohol, glycerin, water. This mixture is then put through a vacuum chamber at low temperatures to evaporate as much liquid as possible. The oily remains are left behind. This mixture is too sticky to put in capsules. Instead, it is mixed together with dried, ground Taheebo Bark. Due to its high concentration of active components, it is said that one capsule will make six cups of tea. This could explain why different taheebo products and extracts have different results. It is legal for a capsule to be filled with bark dust, and called "Taheebo Capsules". However, it's illegal to call the capsule an extract.

How much taheebo a person consumes depends on the purpose. One should not drink more than

2 cups of tea per day if they are drinking it for their daily health maintenance. For those who are using it as a cure for a specific condition, eight or more cups of tea should not be drunk. It has a mild sweet taste and is usually consumed as is. Artificial sweeteners should be avoided if the tea is being used to combat cancer or for diabetics. The tea should only be sweetened with honey, molasses, or maple syrup. These sweeteners contain healthy anti-oxidants. Blueberries can be added to the tea for adults. It has a mild flavor that will quickly adapt to the taste of the fruit.

Chapter 20: Herbalism Plants

Detoxifications and cleansings vary depending on the type of fasting, but it is better to have some of the cleansing herbs in your fasting. If you do decide to go on a water fast for a whole week, then all you need is water and the cleansing herbs in tea.

Cascara Sagrada

It is a shrub that most people know as a "dietary supplements" and was therefore allowed to sell in pharmacies as an OTC drug. However, FDA declared in 2002 that it does not meet the criteria to be sold under the OTC and prescription drugs. The Cascara Sagrada's bark, or dietary supplement, had been used for constipation before 2002. It is a bitterless extract that can be used to flavor foods. This is one of the best things about this shrub.

Rhubarb Root

It is the underground stem and root (or rhizome) from the Rhubarb plant. Traditional Chinese people used the root of the plant as a medicine to treat various digestive disorders, such as stomach pain, constipation (dysmenorrhea), diarrhea and swelling of the pancreas. The stems can be used to flavor great recipes or make delicious pies. The chemical composition of Rhubarb root such as fiber makes it a potent herbal laxative. It can reduce swelling, cure cold sores, improve the tone, health, and function of the digestive tract.

Prodigiosa

It is also known to be called the 'Brickellia Grandiflora herb. It is a daisy-family flowering plant/shrub and is native to California, Mexico and California. These plants/shrubs are used in Mexico to treat symptoms such as diarrhea, diabetes and stomach pain. Prodigiosa has been shown to be an antioxidant. The plant contains chemical compounds that stimulate the pancreatic and lower blood sugar levels. They also aid in digestion and the absorption of fat from the gallbladder.

This improves the healthiness of your stomach digestive system.

Burdock Root

It is the root a Burdock tree, which is widely distributed around the globe. Burdock has many important features. Its root can be eaten as food or medicine, and the seed and leaves can be used for medical purposes. People believe that burdock oral intake can increase the flow and elimination of germs, cleanse blood, treat or prevent cancer, joint pain, nausea, vomiting, anorexia. This plant is not only good for treating and preventing skin conditions like psoriasis and acne. Burdock helps to improve sex drive (libido), lower high blood pressure and cleanse the liver, lymphatic and liver.

Dandelion

It is a common flowering plant. Also known as "Taraxacum Officinale", it is native Europe. It is common to find it in the northern hemisphere, where it thrives in milder climates. These flowering plants are used to treat swelling and inflammation of the pancreas, tonsils, cancer, tonsils, tonsillitis, acne, bladder or urinary tract, digestive, as well as liver disorders. Dandelion is rich in vitamin (A-B, C, C and E), mineral (iron potassium, magnesium, calcium and magnesium), and other compounds (Polyphenols. Chicoric. Chlorogenic acid. It dissolves kidney stones, prevents and treats diabetes, and helps with liver and urinary issues. It also contains chemicals which may increase urine production. This aids in cleansing the bladder and prevents crystals from forming.

Elderberry

It is also known under the name Sambucusnigra, European elderberry, or black elder. It is a native European flowering plant and belongs to the Adoxaceae Family. These flowering plant are very common in Europe, as well as many other places around the world. This plant can reach up to 9 meters. The elderflower is a tall plant that can grow to 30 feet. Elderberry leaves are used for pain relief, inflammation, swelling and to increase urine production. The bark can be used as a laxative or diuretic as well as to induce vomiting.

Guaco

It is also known under the following names: Guace or Vedolin, Cepu, Bejuco de finca and Liane Francois. Cipo caatinga is another name. This climbing plant contains many minerals and compound. It is a member of the Asteraceae species and Asteraceae families. Its leaf is both medicinal and nutritious.

Mullein

It is a flavourful beverage plant also known as "Aaron's Rod", Candlewick, American Mullein and Denseflower Mollein. Candleflower, European or Orange Mullein are all other names. This flavorful beverage plant has been used to treat many illnesses, including asthma, lung disease, colds, chronic coughs and gastrointestinal bleeding.

Natural Herbal Tea

Alfredo Brownman or Dr. Sebi, a Honduran herbalist, said that it is important for the body to be cleansed and detoxified by consistent use of natural botanical remedies.

While natural remedies and herbs are an important part of your journey to greater health, it is also important to remember to adjust your eating habits according to the recommended foods list.

As we've seen, a plant-based nutritional system is vital for healthy eating. However, plants aren't limited to fruits and vegetables. In fact, many herbs have an alkaline effect. We must understand the importance of plants for our health. Their healing effects can reverse and prevent many diseases.

The ancient practice of herbal medicine is very old. It involves a number of healing techniques based upon plants. Modern medicine also recognizes the extraordinary properties many plants have and uses them as common medications.

Most of their macronutrients can be assumed in a completely natural manner by infusions. This is why we shouldn't ignore them in our alkaline food. Chamomile, a very well-known and loved plant, is one of my favorites. Although many people drink it for relaxation or sleeping, they don't realize its important alkaline properties. When stressed or anxious, the body makes more acid. So chamomile tea is a relaxing way to help your body balance its pH.

Chamomile has a powerful anti-inflammatory effect.

Alfalfa

It is also known by the name Lucerne. It is a lesser-known herb that contains a high amount of nutrients. Its name means "Father of All Foods" and it is rich in vitamins, minerals, protein, essential amino acids, and other nutrients. It is able to not only alkalize, but also resets your metabolism. This will help you avoid many common diseases. Here are some details:

Lower the cholesterol

Increase the functionality of your immune system

Cleanse your blood

Support digestion

Alleviate allergic reactions

All forms of arthritis treated

Migraine and headache relief

Alfalfa tea should always be consumed every day. If you're not a fan of its mild flavor, you can mix it with another flavored beverage. This herb is also available in capsules. You can take this herb in capsules, or you could use it as a whole. This herb is the key to an amazing and healthy life.

Dandelion can be used as an alkaline herb in a tea or as part of a salad. It has potent Antioxidants and is an effective treatment for kidney stones.

Dandelion is rich in vitamin A and folic Acid, which can be affected by heat. For this reason, it should be eaten fresh as a vegetable and used to make delicious salads with other vegetables. Dandelion can be easily grown in your garden or fields, and is therefore very inexpensive. You should consider adding it to your daily healthy diet.

Red Clover

One of the most popular medicinal herb teas is one that's based on red clover. It is high in antioxidants and contains isoflavones. They are used for cancer prevention as well as indigestion, asthma, and the treatment of bronchitis. Red clover can be used by women to promote female reproductive health. It may also reduce breast cancer risk.

There are many herbs that are very undervalued. Many people assume that their sole purpose is to add flavor and color to our dishes. However, it's not true. Basil, parsley, cilantro, oregano and sage are all examples.

Parsley

Parsley is an herbal. Parsley is a herb. Its root, seed, as well as the leaf, can be used in medicine.

People take it orally for high blood pressure, constipation (for kidney stones), gastrointestinal disorders, constipation.

No one knows that parsley has higher levels of vitamin C than oranges. The parsley has a high level of vitamin K and iron.

Basil

It releases high amounts eugenol in our bodies, which is a powerful antioxidant. Oregano also contains high levels of the anti-inflammatory agent free-radical fighting agents. There are many alkaline herbs you can use to create excellent infusions.

Laurel

It works well against respiratory diseases like cough, bronchitis or pharyngitis. It has positive effects on arteriosclerosis treatment and vascular problems. Essential oil also has antibacterial properties and antitussive effects.

Chapter 21: Burns And Irritation

Burns can occur from direct contact of body parts with hot liquid, steam, heat, gases, fire, electricity, and chemicals.

Children and the elderly are most vulnerable and may require hospitalization even though only a small amount of their condition is present.

You should immediately seek medical attention in serious cases.

REMEDIES

It has been long used externally to soothe burns, and other types of sores by combining beetroot with olive oil.

The best treatment for burns is to use a raw potato that has been pulverized or scraped into a pulp.

GASTRITIS

Gastritis is an irritation or erosion of the stomach's skin. It can happen either abruptly or slowly. The causes include alcoholism, stress, chronic sickness, excessive drinking, stress, chronic vomiting, aspirin, anti-inflammatory drugs, aspirin, and infections by bacteria and viruses.

There are many symptoms, and some people may not have any symptoms. Common symptoms include abdominal pains. Extreme cases can include nausea, vomiting blood, stomach ache, stomach gnawing, or nausea between meals. Gastritis can also cause loss of appetite.

Gastritis may lead to ulcers. In extreme cases, severe blood loss can lead in to stomach cancer.

REMEDIES

The consumption of bananas is helpful for patients suffering from gastritis. It not only helps to reduce the inflammation in your intestines, but it also has very few waste materials that can cause irritation.

HEADACHES

A headache can be described as pain in one or several areas of the head. Sometimes, it may even reach the neck. Headaches occur in different ways. They may affect one or both the head. Sometimes, the pain is concentrated at a specific point. Other times it is spread over the entire head.

A headache can vary in intensity depending on what is causing it. It can happen suddenly or slowly and can last between a few seconds and several days.

Although most headaches are temporary due to fatigue, they could also be symptoms of an underlying illness. They are uncomfortable, can make it difficult for sufferers to focus on tasks and can cause severe pain.

REMEDIES

To ease headaches due to fatigue, you can make a hot tea with lavender and water.

It is believed that a drink consisting of half a pint water and a tablespoonful home-made marmalade, can provide relief for pains in the head and neuralgia.

HEMORRHOIDS

Hemorrhoids also known as pimples are inflamed or swollen veins found in the lower part of the rectum and the anal canal. These are often painful and can result from many factors such as increased pressure in the veins during pregnancy or straining during bowel movements. The anal canal can also be stressed by constipation, diarrhea, and other factors.

There are typically two types: external and internal hemorhoids.

Extern: These are found under the skin surrounding the anus. Here blood may pool and form a painful, hard lump. After straining to pass stool, you might notice blood stains on tissue paper. It is also known by the name clotted (or thrombosed) hemorhoid.

Rectal bleeding: This is the most common symptom. A normal bowel movement may be followed by red flashes in the tissue paper and/or red blood in your toilet bowl.

The symptoms of internal hemorhoids include skin irritation, pain, skin itching, itching and oozing.

If symptoms persist or they occur when you are suffering from another condition, like constipation or diarrhea, seek professional medical advice.

REMEDIES

One traditional remedy is to boil the elder leaves and add olive oil. This mixture is used when it is warm to alleviate symptoms. It can also be used as a second treatment.

INDIGESTION

Indigestion, also known as dyspepsia, can affect all ages and denotes feeling full. It is also called dyspepsia. This condition is usually experienced after heavy meals and overeating. Indigestion affects the stomach and upper belly.

It is caused by eating spicy and fatty foods, stomach problems, irritable stool syndrome, stomach infection, thyroid disease, stomach cancer, and rare cases, stomach cancer.

Indigestion could have some negative effects on your body that may cause discomfort in your stomach. These symptoms include abdominal pain, bloating and vomiting.

Some medications, such as oral contraceptives or aspirin can cause indigestion. Poor eating habits and stress are also causes of indigestion.

REMEDIES

Celery is a traditional remedy for indigestion symptoms. It can be eaten raw, steamed, and in soup.

INSOMNIA

Adults require six to eight hours sleep per night. In order to avoid sleeplessness and insomnia, many people are forced to sleep less than they should. While some people are able to get more sleep than they need due to being busy, others suffer from insomnia because of factors such as stress, illness and environmental conditions, like noise or diet. Most people experience insomnia due to severe illnesses like toothaches, migraines, fractures, stomachaches, and other types of pain.

Even though insomnia does not cause any serious health issues, it can be a problem. It can affect mental alertness, productivity, and vulnerability to illnesses like cold and flu.

REMEDIES

Lettuce is a traditional favorite for its sedative qualities and easy digestion.

Another traditional remedy is to drink onion juice, which is believed can induce sleep.

Chapter 22: Dash Diet Recipes

Breakfast Recipes

Banana Nut Pancakes

Ingredients:

1 cup whole grain flour

2 teaspoons baking flour

1/4 teaspoon cinnamon

1/4 teaspoon salt

1 large banana peeled and mashed

1 cup 1-percent milk

3 large eggs whites

2 teaspoons olive oil

1 teaspoon vanilla extract

2 tablespoons walnuts chopped

Cooking spray

Directions:

Step 1 - In a large bowl combine all the dry ingredients.

Step 2 - In a medium bowl combine the egg whites with milk, mashed bananas oil, vanilla extract, and milk. Continue to beat the mixture until it becomes smooth.

Step 3 - Add the wet ingredient mix to the dry mix. Use a spoon to mix until there are no dry spots. Don't overmix, as this can lead to pancakes that are not fluffy enough.

Step 4 - Lightly spray a large skillet liberally with cooking spray. Place the skillet on the heat-proof plate. Allow the skillet to warm.

Step 5 - Pour 1/4 cup of the batter onto a skillet. Cook until bubbles start to form and edges are set. Flip the pancake on its side and cook the other end.

Step 6 - Repeat step 5 using the rest of the pancake batter. Serve warm and top with non-fat yogurt

Mini Egg Omelets made with cheese and broccoli

Ingredients:

4 whole large eggs

1 cup of egg whites

4 cups broccoli stems

1/4 cup grated Parmigiano-Reggiano cheese

1/4 cup cheddar cheese reduced fat

1 tablespoon olive Oil

Salt and pepper

Cooking spray

Directions:

Step 1 - Preheat the oven to 350°F

Step 2 - Steam the broccoli for 7 minutes in a little bit of water. Once cooked, mash the brocolli into small pieces.

Step 3 - Drizzle olive oil all over the broccoli. Salt and pepper to suit your taste. Stir until well mixed.

Step 4 - Spray a muffin tray with cooking spray. Then, pour the broccoli mixture into a muffin tin. Make sure to evenly distribute the mixture. Now, set the ingredients aside.

Step 5: Mix the eggs, egg yolks and parmesan in a medium bowl. Salt and pepper to suit your taste.

Step 6 - Pour the egg mixture onto the broccoli mixture-filled muffin cups. Each muffin tin must be filled to about 3/4.

Step 7 - Top the muffin tin with the shredded cheese. The muffin tin should be placed in the oven for approximately 20 minutes.

Step 8 - Serve warm with a fruit salsa

Flax Banana Yogurt breakfast muffins

Ingredients:

1 cup rolled Oats, old-fashioned

1 cup whole grain flour

2 tablespoons ground flaxseed

1 teaspoon baking powder

3 large bananas, peeled.

1/4 cup brown Sugar

1/4 cup applesauce, unsweetened

2 teaspoons vanilla essence

Directions:

Step 1: Preheat your oven to 350°F. Spray the muffin tins or use a baking spray to line the cups.

Step 2: In another bowl, mix the flour, baking soda, flaxseed, and oats together.

Step 3: Combine yogurt, bananas sugar, vanilla extract, and applesauce in a separate bowl.

Step 4 - Carefully mix the dry ingredients and the wet ingredients. Mix the ingredients until combined. The batter should not be too crumbly. Do not overmix.

Step 5 - Divide the batter evenly among the muffin tins. Bake for 20 to 25 minutes. When a toothpick inserted between the muffins comes out cleanly, it is time to turn the oven off.

Very Berry Muesli

Ingredients:

1 cup old-fashioned roll oats

1 cup fruit yogurt

1/2 cup 1-percent milk

1/2 cup dried fruit (such as dates, raisins, or Apricots)

1/2 cup frozen blueberries

1/2 cup chopped apple

1/4 cup chopped walnuts, chopped.

Directions:

Step 1: In large bowl, mix the yogurt, milk, and oatmeal together.

Step 2 - Cover the bowl with plastic wrap, and let it rest in the fridge between 6 and 12 hours.

Step 3 - Stir in the blueberries, apples, and dried fruit.

Step 4 - Place the muesli on a plate and add a little chopped and toasted walnuts to the top.

Lunch Recipes

Panini of Swiss and Apple

Ingredients:

8 slices of whole-grain bread

2 slices of thinly sliced crisp apples

1/4 cup non-fat honey mustard

6 ounces low fat Swiss cheese, sliced thin

1 cup arugula Leaves

Cooking spray

Directions:

Step 1 - Heat a Panini pressing on medium heat. Nonstick skillets will also work, even if you don't have a Panini presse.

Step 2: As the skillet heats, drizzle the honey mustard lightly onto each slice.

Step 3 - Layer the Swiss cheese, apple slices, and the arugula on 4 of the bread slices. Place the remaining bread slices on top.

Step 4 - Spray the Panini or skillet with cooking oil.

Step 5 - Place one sandwich in the Panini pressing and grill for around 3 to 5. You want the cheese to melt and the bread to toast.

Step 6 - Repeat step 5 with all three sandwiches. Serve warm.

Southwest Style Rice Bowl

Ingredients:

1 cup chopped vegetables

1 teaspoon vegetable oils

1 cup cooked meat, chopped, shredded or diced

1 cup brown rice cooked

4 tablespoons salsa

2 tablespoons sour Cream, Low Fat

2 tablespoons shredded Cheese

Directions:

Step 1 - Heat the oil in an ovenproof skillet.

Step 2 - Place the vegetables into a skillet.

Step 3 - Add the rice and cooked meats to the skillet. Stir until everything is well heated.

Step 4 - Remove the mixture from the heat and divide into two bowls

Step 5 - Top the mixture with cheese and salsa. Serve warm.

Mayo-Less Tuna Salad

Ingredients:

5 ounce can light tuna in water, drained

1 tablespoon of red wine vinegar

1 tablespoon extra virgin olive oils

1/4 cup chopped green onion tops

2 cups arugula

1 cup cooked pasta

1 tablespoon parmesan cheese freshly shaved

Black pepper

Directions:

Step 1 - Drain the tuna. Toss the tuna in oil.

Step 2 - Add the vinegar, onion tops and cooked pasta. Mix until well combined.

Step 3: Divide your mixture between 2 plates. Sprinkle each portion with black pepper, parmesan, and a little bit of salt. Serve immediately

Sandwiches of Turkey, Cheese, and Pear

Ingredients:

2 slices of multi-grain sandwich bread or rye

2 teaspoon Dijon-style mustard

2 slices of reduced sodium smoked or cooked turkey

1 pear, cored.

1/4 cup shredded low-fat mozzarella cheese

Ground black pepper

Directions:

Step 1 - Spread 1 teaspoon mustard onto each slice of bread

Step 2: Place 1 slice each of turkey on each slice. Place the pear pieces on top. Sprinkle 2 tablespoons of cheese over the turkey.

Step 3 - Broil for around 2 to 3-minutes, or until the pears/turkey are warm and cheese has melted.

Step 4 - Cut the sandwich in half. Serve the sandwich open-faced.

Here are some dinner recipes

Stir Fry of Chicken and Cabbage

Ingredients:

3 chicken breast halves

1 teaspoon olive oil or vegetable oil

3 cups shredded red cabbage

1 tablespoon cornstarch

1/4 teaspoon garlic powder

1/2 teaspoon ground ginger

1 tablespoon soya sauce, low-sodium

1/2 cup water

Directions:

Step 1 - Pour the vegetable oil and olive oil into a pan. Place on the stove and heat it to medium-high heat. Heat the oil.

Step 2 - Heat the oil. Cut the breasts of chicken into strips. Put the strips into the hot oil and fry. Then turn the strips around and fry them until golden brown. Continue turning the chicken over until it is fully cooked.

Step 3 - Add the cabbage to a skillet. Let the cabbage cook until tender. This takes about 2 minutes.

Step 4 - In a small bowl combine the cornstarch powder, garlic powder, and ground ginger. Add the soy sauce to the water. Mix until smooth.

Step 5 - Add the sauce to chicken and cabbage mixture. Cook the chicken for about 20 minutes or until the sauce is thickening.

Step 6 - Serve warm

Quick 5-Ingredient Chili

Ingredients:

1/2 pound ground meat, 95 percent lean

1/2 medium onion chopped

1 can (14.5 ounces), diced tomatoes containing liquid

1 can (15.5 ounces), kidney bean, drained

1 1/2 cups chili powder

Directions:

Step 1: Brown the meat and onions together in a large saucepan.

Step 2 - Drain the fat off the meat. Place the meat in the skillet.

Step 3 - Add the beans, chili powder, tomatoes. Reduce the heat down to low. Cover the skillet, and cook for about 10 min.

Step 4 - Serve hot

Lean Meat Cheeseburgers

Ingredients:

1 pound ground beef, 95 percent lean

2 tablespoons quick cooking oats

1/2 teaspoon steak seasoning combination

4 slices cheese, low-fat

4 whole wheat or seeded burger buns

Toppings (optional), such as lettuce leaves and tomato slices

Directions:

Step 1 - Place the oats and water in a Ziplock bag. Seal the bag tightly and get rid of any excess air. Use a rolling mill to grind the oats until they are fine.

Step 2 - Place the chopped oats in a large bowl. Add the ground meat and steak seasoning. Mix all ingredients together with your hands. The mixture should be formed into four patties, each about 1/2 inch thick.

Step 3 - Place the hamburger patties on a grill. Grill until done. The meat can be horizontally inserted with a thermometer. The hamburgers can be grilled when the internal temperature reaches 160°F.

Step 4 - Layer your toppings and meats on the bottom part of the hamburger bun. Cover the top half of the bun.

Grilled Salmon and Dill Sauce

Ingredients:

2 pounds salmon steaks

1 cup plain yogurt, sugar-free

2 teaspoon minced fresh dill

1/4 cup chopped scallions

1 teaspoon capers

1 teaspoon chives, minced

2 teaspoons minced parsley

1 tablespoon olive Oil

Directions:

Step 1: In small bowl, mix yogurt, dill and parsley. Keep the sides aside.

Step 2 - Spray the grill racks and cookware with nonstick spray.

Step 3: Season each salmon steak with olive oils. Each steak should be grilled for 4 minutes on each side, using medium or hot coals. The salmon steaks should be done when the salmon has flakes easily with a knife.

Step 4 - Serve the salmon steaks and the dill sauce side by side

Macaroni made with Whole Wheat Macaroni and Light Cheddar

Ingredients:

3/4 pound Whole Wheat elbow macaroni

2 cups Panko breadcrumbs

3 butter, unsalted

1/3 cup + 1 1/2 cups shredded cheddar cheese, reduced-fat

2 tablespoons fresh rosemary

3 tablespoons all-purpose flour

2 3/4 cups fatfree milk

1 cup chicken stock, low-sodium

2 teaspoons Dijon mustard

1/4 teaspoon ground black Pepper

Directions:

Step 1: Heat the oven to 400°F. Butter a 3-quart shallow baking dish. Move to the side for now.

Step 2 - Fill a large pan with water until it is about 3/4 full. Cook the macaroni in a large pot until they are al dente. Drain the water, and let cool on the side.

Step 3 - In a large skillet, melt the butter. Add the breadcrumbs. Add the black pepper to the butter and stir the breadcrumbs until they turn golden brown. Allow to cool. Stir in 1/3 cup cheddar cheese.

Step 4 - Melt the butter in a large saucepan over medium heat. Mix in the flour. Continue stirring for three minutes. Mix in the milk, and bring to boil. Whisk constantly. Reduce the heat and simmer, stirring occasionally for approximately 3 minutes. Stir in 1 1/2 cups cheddar cheese. Add the thyme. Take off the heat.

Step 5: Mix the drained pasta, sauce, and chicken broth together in a large mixing bowl.

Step 6 - Pour the mixture into a baking dish. Sprinkle the cheese mixture, breadcrumbs, and even the macaroni evenly.

Step 7 - Bake the baking dish for 20-25 mins.

Step 8 - Remove the oven from the heat and allow to cool.

Dessert Recipes

Blueberry Bling

Ingredients:

3 cups blueberries frozen or fresh

2 teaspoons softened margarine or butter (softened, not melted)

1 cup brown sugar

1 tablespoon all purpose flour

1/2 cup rolled, oats

1/2 teaspoon cinnamon

Directions:

Step 1 - Preheat oven to 350°F

Step 2 - While the oven preheats, wash and drain your blueberries.

Step 3 - Place the blueberries cleaned in a 9 inch pie plate

Step 4 - Use a spoon to combine the soft butter or margarine with brown sugar, flour, oatmeal, and cinnamon.

Step 5 - Sprinkle the mixture over the blueberries

Step 6 - Place the pie plate in the oven and bake for 25 min

Step 7 - Serve warm

Milk Chocolate Pudding

Ingredients:

2 tablespoons cocoa butter

3 tablespoons cornstarch

2 tablespoons sugar

1/8 teaspoon salt

2 cups nonfat milk

1/3 cup chocolate chips

1/2 teaspoon vanilla extract

Directions:

Step 1: In medium saucepan, mix the cocoa powder, cornstarch and sugar. Mix until everything is well mixed.

Step 2 - Add the milk to a saucepan and place it on the stove. Stir frequently and heat on medium.

Continue stirring the mixture and heating it until it thickens and bubbles.

Step 3 - Remove the saucepan from the heat. Stir in the vanilla bean and chocolate chips. Keep stirring until chocolate chips are melted. The pudding should be smooth.

Step 4 - Divide the pudding among 4 plates or 1 large bowl. Put the pudding in the refrigerator and allow it to chill for at least two hours.

Simple Apples and Cream Shake

Ingredients:

1 cup unsweetened applesauce

2 cups vanilla ice cream, low-fat

1/4 teaspoon ground cinnamon, apple pie spice, or

1 cup skim milk, fat free

Directions:

Step 1 - Place the ice cream mixture, applesauce and apple spice of ground ginger in a blender. Blend until smooth.

Step 2 - Pour the skimmed cream into the blender. Blend once more until smooth.

Step 3 - Pour the shake in glasses. Sprinkle with cinnamon or additional apple pie spice, if you wish.

Step 4 - Serve immediately

Tip - You can replace low-fat frozen ice cream with low-fat vanilla yogurt by adding 1 cup of vanilla yogurt.

Chapter 23: Aromatherapy

Aromatherapy can be more than just a way to have nice aromas around your house. It can also help you feel better.

This chapter examines aromatherapy and alternative medicine. We go back in time and see how and where it was first used, and what it can offer us today.

Aromatherapy explained

Aromatherapy is when oil from a plant is extracted (in certain cases this is done chemically). It is then used to promote wellbeing. The essential oil is the essence of the plant.

Essential oils are known to promote a "better mental state", which can include reducing stress, calming, or having less painful symptoms. There are also essential oils that can be used to relieve physical symptoms. For example, peppermint can be used to ease indigestion; clove oil can be rubbed on sore teeth (but not if there is an abscess); and lavender can be used for burns.

Although it has been proven that essential oils have a positive effect on mental, physical, as well as emotional well-being, their use is still limited.

Aromatherapy can aid in the treatment of many ailments, including: inflammation, disease, pain management, muscle ache, blood circulation, stress and anxiety as well as headaches.

It is believed that there are two types of effects. The aroma's effect on the brain is one, and the body is the other. Aromatherapy does not cure. However, it can help our bodies heal.

Aromatherapy History

Since the beginning records, aromas played an important role in history. Trading was possible because of the high demand for sandalwood and other spices.

It was the hunt for plants that inspired both the Egyptians and the Greeks to travel into central Africa. The Greeks also traveled to distant islands, while the Chinese left the mainland.

Many ancient medicines were based on aromatic plants. At first, the prescribed items contained only herbs that were effective. However, soon these were mixed with magical ingredients. This was either to make the items more visible or to give them a shock factor. No one seems to know if it was because the "doctors" believed these ingredients had real value.

They were used in religious ceremonies.

Hippocrates recommended essential oils. He was ahead of his time and suggested that they should be used for preventative medicine.

Aromatherapy: How do you use it?

Aromatherapy can be described as the use of essential oils to complement or cure scientific treatment.

There are many ways you can reap the benefits aromatherapy has to offer.

This may be a personal way of thinking, such as

In your bath, add oil

Get a massage

Apply oil to your pulse points to maintain a continuous smell

Making a "water spray spray" by diluting an aroma in water and spraying your face with the mist

Add body creams

steam inhalation

It may be located in your home.

You can make your own air fresheners by adding a few drops to a spray-bottle of water and shaking it.

To create room fragrances, scrub the old peach kernels. Then place in a dish with oil and drizzle some oil. To create a whole room scent, coat half of each kernel with silicone. The silicone will prevent oil stains from forming on shelves and carpets.

Oil burners – add a few drops in oil to water.

Reed diffusers – Mix some oil with water in an old bottle of reed to create a therapeutic fragrance

You can also add to potpourri by making your own with pine cones, flower petals, and buds.

Candles: Melt old, unscented candles and add essential oil. Place the candle in a dish or add a light wick.

To eliminate odours in smoke, a blend of rosemary essential Oil, tea tree oils (anti-microbial), or eucalyptus essential oil should suffice. While cooking smells will require peppermint essential and lavender oil, it is possible to get rid of them.

What Each Oil Type Does

There are so many to list, but here are some of the most commonly used.

Cedarwood

This aftershave has a woody smell and is great for men. It's calming and helps to reduce catarrh when inhaled.

Eucalyptus

This steam inhalant has a pine-fresh, citrus-y scent and can be used to reduce the symptoms of headaches. It helps to lessen the pain of headaches.

Ginger

This warm and spicy aroma acts as a tonic.

Rosemary

This pain reliever is anti-bacterial, antiseptic, and pain relief. It cleanses the mind and body, gives you energy, and promotes circulation.

Sandalwood

This oil is considered one of the most valuable essential oils. Its rich, woody aroma lowers blood pressure, and it can be used as a room scent to promote a feeling of well-being.

Ylang Ylang

Ylang Ylang has a strong floral scent that is soothing and calming.

Patchouli

It is anti-fungal and has an earthy fragrance.

Peppermint

Peppermint is good at digestion and is available in drops to inhale. It can also help with bad breath and headaches.

Aromatherapy may have side effects

Every substance is different, so each person will react differently to it. Even though there are not many adverse effects, essential oils can cause some side effects. It is important to understand what the oil does before you buy it.

Side effects from using essential oils to scent your home or skin are usually caused by the oil being ingested. Ask your doctor before you rub or apply essential oils.

Personal Experience

I use essential oils in every area of my home, mostly using peach kernels. I also used a few drops Ylang Ylang for my bath. I added 5-10 drops to the bottle. I believed it would be fine and that no oil would have come out from the tiny hole in my bottle. So, I went to the bath and felt amazing for the next 30 minutes. It was then that I felt weak and couldn't get up. I had to call my partner to get him to drain the water and then lift me onto the mattress. I felt great again after an hour.

This article should not be interpreted as a substitute for expert medical advice. You should consult your physician before taking any steps to improve your health.

Chapter 24: Herbs & Optimal health

We all desire to live a fulfilling and happy life. But, there are many things that get in the way of our reaching these vital goals. Not only does it mean living a healthy lifestyle, but also mental, emotional and spiritual well-being. You can stay healthy physically, mentally, and emotionally by eating healthy. They all have an effect on your overall wellbeing. It is important to consume different types of food (carbohydrates as well as fats and protein) but they won't make you healthier. Natural remedies are not enough. You need to be able to use other natural remedies to avoid getting sick from artificial compounds. Many people have used herbs for centuries to treat, cure and prevent illness. It is a good idea to learn how to keep your body healthy by using different herbs. Which herbs can you use for staying healthy?

Different herbs can be used for health and general well-being. Each herb has a different method of preparation and application.

Some key benefits of using herbs include:

*Herbs can be used repeatedly and have low side effect rates, are safe, and natural.

*Herbs may be effective in the treatment of chronic conditions that cannot be treated by traditional medicine.

*Herbs are easily affordable because they are readily available.

*Herbs are safe from toxic chemicals that can cause harm to the body.

How to Use Herbs

Before we start to discuss the many herbs you can use to improve your health, it is important that you take a look around at all the ways you can use herbs. Keep in mind that the type of herb you wish to use will also determine how it should be used.

Herbal Teas

Making herbal teas is one way to use herbs. Herbal teas can be made quickly and are very effective. There are three main ways of making tea. Decoction, infusion and brewing are all options. We will be discussing these different ways to make herbal teas.

Herbal Infusions

Infusions are made mostly from the leaves and flowers of plants. You should steep delicate parts rather than boil them to unlock their healing properties.

Herbal Decoctions

Decoctions can be made from boiling the herb. This is simply a way to boil the herbs. The herb will determine how long it takes to boil and how much water you use.

Herbal Brews

This simply refers to the fermentation of an infusion or decoction.

Herbal Tinctures

Tinctures simply contain concentrated liquid extracts. They are highly potent so they can only be consumed in very small amounts. Tinctures should be diluted with juice or warm water. You can use 1/2 to 1 teaspoon per day for chronic problems. 1/4 to 1/2 teaspoon per 60 minutes is sufficient for acute problems.

While most tinctures are made with alcohol as the main solvent, there is very little alcohol in them. ACV and vegetable glycerin may be used instead. We'll be looking at the simple steps involved in making tinctures.

1. Take the chopped herbs and place them in a jar. Then, pour the solvent on top. Use vinegar before heating it. Vegetable glycerin should be diluted with water before it is used on the herbs. Be sure to pour enough solvent so that the herbs are fully submerged.

2. Keep the jar warm for at least one month. Ensure you shake the jar at least once a day during the maceration period.

3. The stainless-steel strainer should be lined with muslin. After straining the herbs, label the container and rebottle the liquid. This must be kept out from children's reach and stored in a dark area.

Steam Inhale

The herbs can also be boiled in hot water, and you can inhale their steam. This is a great way to clear congestion from the sinuses or chest.

Herbal compresses

The herbs are then held to the skin directly in cold or hot extracts such as tea, tincture or dried form. Poultices work in the same way as compresses. But poultices may be messy because although they have the same components, they are mixed with clay to make a paste or use powdered herbs.

Herb Capsules

Making powdered herbs and capsules involves drying, grinding, and then sifting the herbs to create capsules in powdered tooth powders and body powders.

Now that you are familiar with the various ways herbs can serve you, let us now discuss the different types of herbs that you can use to improve your health.

Chapter 25: Proven Methods To Keep A Young Look

All the latest cosmetic procedures can give you a youthful glow. A facial treatment can be done in just 15 minutes and you will see glowing skin immediately. It is important to maintain a healthy appearance over time without resorting to cosmetic procedures. You must develop a beauty routine to follow for years. Here are some ways to keep your appearance young.

Brighten up your wardrobe

Your wardrobe can say a lot about you. Your wardrobe can speak volumes about your taste, style, and even age. Your wardrobe may be cluttered with boring clothes, sweatshirts and pants, so it's easy to look older than you are. It is now that you need to spice up what you have!

Dressing young is the best way to look young. It doesn't matter if you are older or not. You can still be fashionable and trendy. There are many ways to look younger if you dress up. You just need to explore. You can start by getting rid off those boring black tops and dresses. You don't have to wear funeral attire. You don't have to be overly covered in light-colored clothes. Be able to show some skin and identify your physical assets.

Apply moisturizer and exfoliate

Your skin can look tired from the accumulation of dead skin cells. These are layers that have become darkened over time and must be removed. The body does naturally exfoliate but this can be tedious. You could help with the natural exfoliating process using body scrubs or salts. Exfoliating can cause your body to lose natural moisture so moisturize as soon as you finish.

A moisturizer is an essential step to maintain a youthful appearance of your skin. Dry skin can be patchy and easily irritated by sun exposure. The body is naturally moist, but factors such as sun exposure and stress can dry out your skin. So your skin can stay hydrated at all times, make sure you have a moisturizer!

Release once in a long time

Stress is a major cause of premature aging. While stress is inevitable, it should not be a hindrance to your ability to look and feel younger. Relax and take a breather from the stress. This will help you to deal with all the pressures and strains in life. You deserve it!

Laugh whenever you have the chance

Laugh lines are more important than wrinkles. Laughing makes your body relax, which can make you feel happier and lighter. Science will also show that smiling takes far less facial muscles to do than frowning. This helps to relax your facial muscles. You will look younger and more radiant when you laugh.

Being young isn't just about being young in years. It's also about being young in spirit. Be a person you love and nurture in every aspect of your life. You'll soon see a youthful appearance.

Chapter 26: Essential Herb Oils To Use In Holistic & Naturopathy Spa

Consistency is key for aromatherapy treatments' success. Your personal rituals should be a part of your daily routine. You don't need to use all of the oils. I recommend starting with just 1-3 essential oils. If you are new or unfamiliar with aromatherapy, I suggest that you visit your local natural health/naturopathy store to ask them for essential oils testers.

In order to reap the mental and psychological benefits of essential oils (EO), my teacher once gave me a tip which I still use. It will help guide you, and it will make you more attracted to the oils you find healing. You should still learn a bit about the properties and get some direction and guidance.

This is what this chapter has to offer.

Aromatherapy rules/blended aromatherapy

The following proportions are important to remember:

-Add 5 to 7 drops of essential oils to 15ml of vegetable olive oil (equals 1 tablespoon).

-Add 1 drop of essential oil to 2mls of vegetable oil

Concentrate less on the face if possible, especially if your skin is sensitive.

30-ml vegetable oil (or crème) can be used with 1- 2 drops of essential oils.

It also depends upon the essential oil used. Verbena, a favorite of mine, can be irritating if it's applied on the skin. I typically use only one drop of verbena oil EO in 10 ml vegetable oils. This blend works well for nighttime facial massages. I find it to be nourishing and great for oily skin types like mine. This is my go-to anti-insomnia oil.

Let's take you through the entire army of essential oils for weight-loss (EO).

GRAPEFRUIT EO (citrus x paradisi)

This oil can have many different properties for the mind and body. It does the following:

*Antidepressant

*Antiseptic

*Disinfectant

*Diuretic

*Stimulant

*Tonic

Grapefruit EO:

- It can be used to energize you and increase your metabolism. This is recommended for times of fatigue or exhaustion.

- It curbs cravings and helps prevent binge eating.

- Natural anti-cellulite treatment

- Acts naturally as a diuretic and prevents water from being retained

- Natural remedy for food cravings

- It helps eliminate toxins from your body, and can also relieve hangover symptoms

- Stimulates lymphatic circulation and vein circulation

It has a very positive and energizing effect on me. It's also useful for those suffering from physical and mental exhaustion. Students, athletes, and any active person can use it.

I use 2-3 drops of grapefruit essential oil in 1 tablespoon of VO to calm my nerves.

You can apply it topically (as described in the previous Chapter) or aromatically (inhalation and direct inhalation). As a quick and easy fix, I use this method.

It is known that this oil can increase self-acceptance, selfconfidence, and trust. I guarantee it will put your mood in the right place. It is possible to describe the "good mood" in many different ways. Because everyone is unique, so is each person's emotional reaction to essential oil. I have only mentioned the most common soothing and emotional reactions people experience.

Caution:

*Avoid sunbathing up to 12 hours following use

LEMON EO (Citrus Limon)

Here's another citrus essential oils with many therapeutic properties. Its actions are:

176

*Anti-anemic

*Antimicrobial

*Antirheumatic

*Antitoxic

*Bactericidal

*Depurative

*Diuretic

*Hypotensive

*Tonic

It acts as an effective diuretic, and it prevents water loss. It stimulates white corpuscles and is great for the immune system.

PEPPERMINTEO (Menthapiperita)

Here's another EO that will energize you, and stimulate your metabolism. This is a great EO for hot summers. It provides a refreshing and rejuvenating feeling, and helps to combat fatigue that can be caused by high temperatures.

I personally like the scents created by mixing this oil (e.g., with one of these citrus essential oils) verbena, lemon, orange, bergamot).

It's not only full of healing properties but also acts as:

*Anti-inflammatory

*Cephalic (prevents headaches)

*Vasoconstrictor

*Stomachic

*Antiseptic

It can also be used to soothe migraines, nervous stress, mental fatigue, and other nervous disorders. Its pleasant scent makes me yearn for healthier beverages. I use this oil after a shower in the summer. I typically dilute the oil with organic cream or Aloe Vera Gel. I end my refreshment time with an energizing smoothie. This oil can take over any unhealthy food cravings and laziness.

This oil is very powerful. I recommend you use lower concentrations for full body massages. One tablespoon of your favorite vegetable oil can be sufficient to use 2 drops. You may need to strengthen your blend if you find it too weak. But wait a bit before you apply the blend to your body. If you use this oil for massage, it can cause a loss of coolness.

Use direct inhalation to quickly get relief. Peppermint essential Oil is great for emotional eating prevention.

Precautions:

Use small amounts to avoid irritation of the skin or mucous membranes.

JUNIPER EO (Juniperus communis)

The oil of Juniper EO is a natural, cleansing spa treatment. Juniper EO can be used as:

*Depurative

*Diuretic

*Tonic

For regular massage, this oil is essential if you wish to prevent the accumulation of toxins and gout.

It has a soothing, woody aroma that is great for people who don't like strong fragrances.

My experience is that it gives immediate relief for tired, heavy legs. This feeling usually occurs when you sit too much or are standing for too long. Based on my personal experience, if you feel this way, you will want to get home, eat, and maybe even eat fast food.

It's not something I would recommend, so I suggest that you use juniper essential oil to massage your body after a shower. This is how you can start to feel the soothing effects of juniper essential oil on a physical level. You will also be able move your body for up to 15 minutes and feel great for the rest of your day.).

Inhaling, steaming, or directly with the oil will have a positive impact on your nervous systems. This oil is great for any anxiety-related condition.

It can also be used for other purposes, if you decide to buy this oil.

*Skin & hair care (acne/hair-loss and oily complexions) you can simply massage your scalp and apply the treatment (always dilute, as explained in the previous chapter).

*Immune system: It helps to relieve colds, flu, or other infections. I've used it to massage my throat and chest when I was suffering from the flu. It provided relief that didn't require me to use any other medications. It helped me to sleep better when I was ill.

SWEET ORANGE EO (Citrus sinensis)

I cannot have enough of citrus oils.

I am certain that this oil is an important part of our daily lives.

I use it daily to keep my body healthy, vital, and slim. Holistic health will always produce a balanced body.).

It acts as a weight-loss essential oil by stimulating the lymphatic, digestive and immune systems. The lymphatic system helps eliminate toxins and prevents them from building up in the body. It is also essential to function properly in order for our immune system to be healthy. When the lymphatic system does not function properly, there are a number of health problems. They may be mistaken for a cosmetic issue, like cellulite or swelling. They are symptoms of a deeper problem that needs to be addressed.

You can take simple steps to take better care your lymphatic system.

-Healthy, balanced nutrition (I advocate an alkaline diet).

-Regular exercise (this is the only way to go!)

-Request a lymphatic massage. A regular massage with essential oils in plain or diluted form, such as Citrus sinesis, is a good idea.

English: Sweet Orange essential oil.

The detoxifying properties of the herb are not only beneficial on a physical level but also help to calm your nervous system. As you will see, both from personal experience and after reading the rest of my blog, the nervous and digestive systems, along with your conscious choices about food, and any actions you take, are interconnected.

Sweet Orange essential oil is a great choice for nervous system support. It is great at reducing stress and nervous tension. I use it to get better sleep. Use this to help you sleep like a baby. Choose how you feel and balance your emotions!

Summarising, multifunctional oil acts as a natural and effective lymphatic drainage. It can also fight water retention.

Simply add a few drops to a vegetable oil base and massage your skin. You can also inhale the incredible, relaxing aroma. It improves sleep quality and combats stress.

There are many other uses for oil you can make if it is not your first choice:

*Skincare is a natural treatment for oily skin

*Respiratory system- Provides relief for flu, bronchitis, or cold symptoms

*Immune system: It helps stimulate the lymphatics system. If used frequently, it can help prevent infections and increase energy levels.

Precautions: Avoid direct sun exposure for upto 10-12 hours

Conclusion

We've seen how honey can provide a multitude of wonderful benefits. You'll notice a significant improvement in your health, and you'll be happy that honey has been added to your diet.

We are taught that foods found in nature can be healthier than processed foods.

Yes, it's possible to go to a trusted supermarket today and purchase your first week's honey. You will be so glad you did. Over time, you'll forget everything about sugar. You'll wonder why so many people have become so dependent on it. If you truly need to be dependent on anything, let it be honey.

www.ingramcontent.com/pod-product-compliance
Lightning Source LLC
Chambersburg PA
CBHW060330030426
42336CB00011B/1280